THIS GUIDE BELONGS TO:

____

____

____

May "The Resilient Dancer" be the spark that fuels your love for dance, reminding you that resilience is the heartbeat of your journey. You are so much more than the outcome of any practice or performance; you are the embodiment of dedication, the essence of grace under pressure, and a living testament to the breathtaking beauty that unfolds when strength and artistry come together. Here's to dancing with your whole being, embracing every step of your journey with unwavering courage, and celebrating the remarkable dancer you are destined to become.

www.myballetworld.com

How To Get the Most Out of This Guide

We recommend reading one tool at a time and applying the tips and exercises for a month in your life and your training. This way you will get the benefits of practicing the tools, rather than just reading the theory.

Of course you can also read through the guide first, choose the tools you need most, and apply them in your daily routine.

However you choose to use this guide, there is one thing that is guaranteed: your ballet life will never be the same again!

You will start to act in a more caring and loving way towards yourself, and that alone will create exponential growth in your health and happiness.

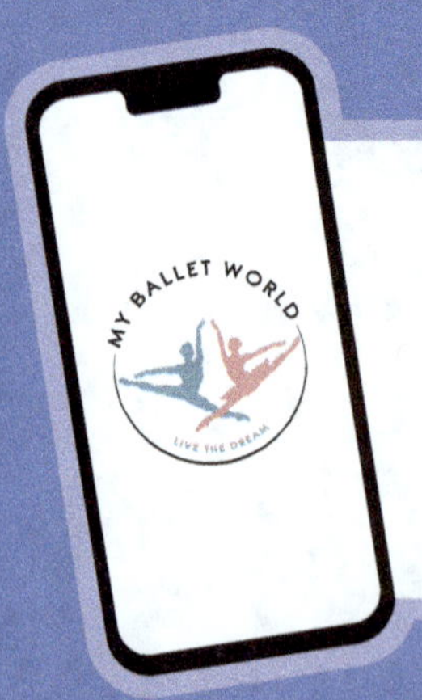

Download the
My Ballet World App
for meditations tailored specifically to the unique needs of ballet dancers.

When we were doing the research for this guide, we were surprised at how few studies and useful tools were out there that were aimed specifically for dancers.

In the best case, dancers are treated only as athletes by the scientific community and as a result, the unique challenges a ballet dancer faces are totally underestimated.

This is what motivated us to create **The Resilient Ballet Dancer Guide**.

Our aim is to offer dancers around the world all the tools necessary to achieve great dancing performance but also stay healthy and happy along the way.

Ballet has an expiry date, and the worst thing that can happen to a dancer is to not be able to enjoy every moment of this magical art because of a bad injury or negative mental state.

This guide will help you grow exponentially as a dancer BUT ALSO stay healthy and happy. We have created this guide with the unique characteristics of a ballet dancer in mind, and we address the unique challenges that dancers face every day.

In this guide, we will cover:

Setting goals

Dealing with perfectionism

Positive self-talk

Visualization for dancers

Fruitful failure

Non-stop motivation

The comparison trap

Mindfulness for dancers

Building confidence

Making stress your best friend

Avoiding injuries

Your personal toolkit for success

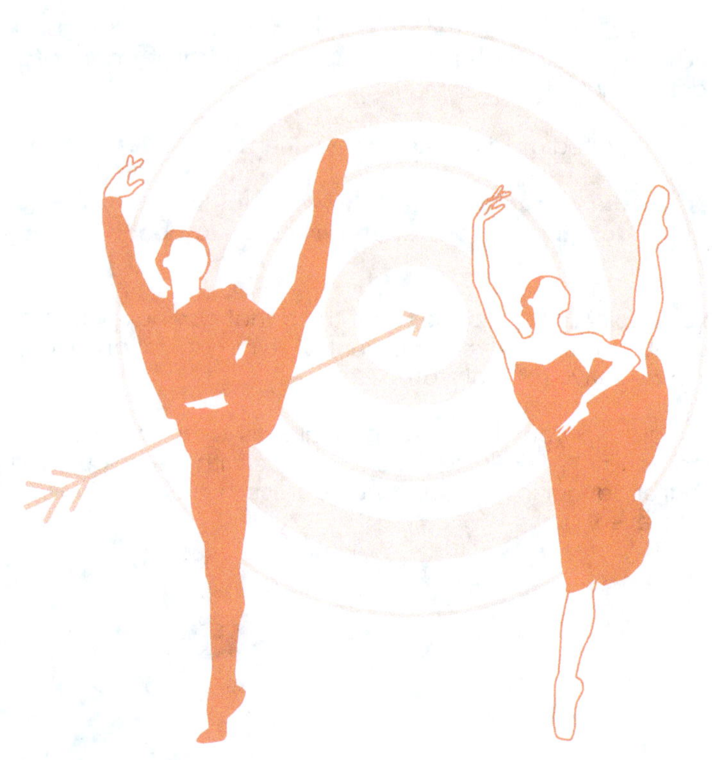

Setting Goals

Your Roadmap to Unfolding Ballet Brilliance

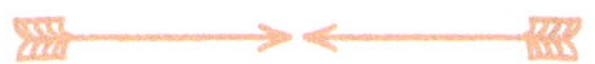

The journey towards every desire and dream you have as a dancer can be exciting and magical, but it's not always going to be a smooth road. You already know that difficult times, difficult emotions, and obstacles often arise.

Goal setting gives you a better sense of direction, and provides you with a road map to follow in order to achieve your dance dream.

Essentially, goal setting is a mental training technique that helps you to identify what you want to achieve and what you will do to get there.

Goal setting is linked with higher motivation, self-esteem, and self-confidence. Research has established a strong connection between goal setting and success.

Goals also help you set clear expectations and new challenges. They give meaning to your actions, helping you strive for higher things. The experience of setting goals, working toward them, and achieving them can give you an amazing sense of confidence and motivation. As a result, you will dream even bigger and achieve more and more.

However, goal setting is not always easy. Sometimes we set goals that are much higher than our level and physical ability, and we may end up disappointed or injured. At times, we set goals that are simplistic and fail to lead us in the right direction.

So let's make it really easy and practical to set your dance goals.

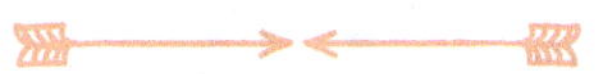

How to Set Goals

Research shows that to give yourself the best chance of achieving a goal, this goal needs to be SMART:

S Specific

M Measurable

A Action-oriented

R Realistic

T Timely

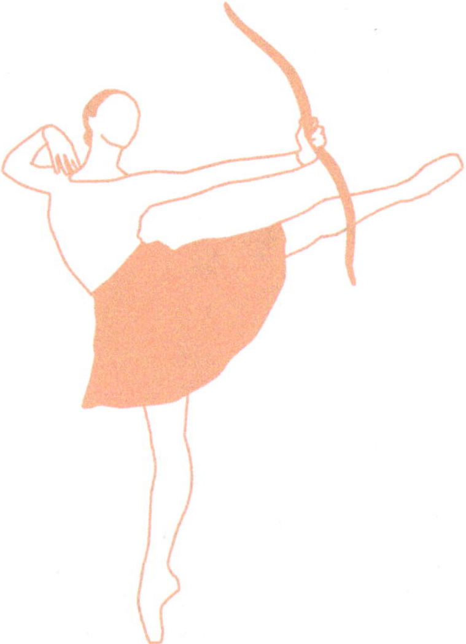

Let's look at this in more detail:

1. Set Specific Goals

Having a vague or generalized idea about your goal isn't efficient at all. Your goal should be clear, specific and detailed.

For instance:

A goal such as "I want to improve my pirouettes" expresses a general desire. But "I want to master a flawless double pirouette ending on a balance" is a specific goal.

A goal such as "I want to improve my sleep" is also something general. But "I want to get an undisturbed eight hours of sleep every night from 23:00 to 07:00" is a specific goal.

2. Set Measurable Goals

Goals must be measurable so you know when you have reached your desired result. What measures of quantity and quality will be used to determine whether your goal has been achieved?

For example:

Goal: "Getting a clear, 90-degree arabesque"

Measures of quantity and quality that you can set:

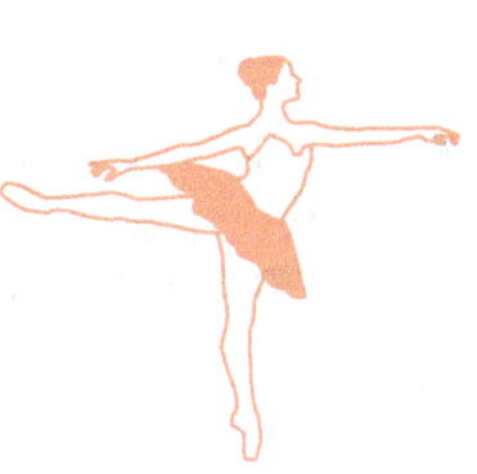

- 90-degree arabesque
- Strong and well turned out supporting leg
- Straight and pointed working leg
- Shoulders down and squared with the rib cage and hips.
- No tension in my neck and arms

This way, you can easily and measurably follow the progress of your goal.

In the above example, it can be really helpful to record yourself in order to gain a clear picture of your current arabesque. Repeat the process every two weeks or month in order to check your progress.

3. Action-oriented Goals

Action-oriented goals require you to outline in detail the steps required to achieve them. This type of goal is more motivating, as it provides you with a clear road map of what you need to do.

Let's continue with the example of the arabesque.

ACTIONS

- I'll ask my teacher for help and guidance
- I'll work on my back strength and flexibility by doing this…
- I'll focus on stretching my hips and spine by doing this…
- I'll acquire pelvic and hip control by doing this exercise…
- I'll book two Pilates classes per week.

Hint: It's also really important to define a particular time in your day when you'll do these specific actions. Otherwise they can easily be forgotten.

4. Set Realistic Goals

Goals need to be challenging, but they also need to be realistic. Therefore, a goal should be defined by your current level and the needs of your body.

Goals need to be challenging, but they also need to be realistic. Therefore, a goal should be defined by your current level and the needs of your body.

For instance, it is unrealistic for your goal to be "master a quadruple pirouette," if you're barely able to do a double pirouette. Instead, your goal should be "get a clean double pirouette," and then a triple, then a quadruple!

If you try to rush to the next level, you are likely to delay the process.

However, you need to find a balance. You don't want to set goals that are too difficult because they will quickly frustrate you and make you want to give up. Similarly, you don't want to set goals that are too easy because it won't challenge you.

Aim to set goals that are both achievable and ambitious. They should be goals that you can obtain through hard work and persistence.

5. Set Time-bound Goals

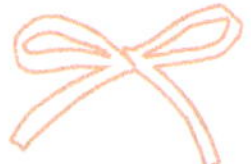

Putting a time limit on your goal is a great way to increase your motivation. A deadline can help you focus and put in the necessary time and energy.

The time limit should be short enough to give you a sense of focus or urgency, but long enough for the goal to be achievable.

Short-term goals typically have a time frame of 3-12 months. Here are some examples:

- Get higher extensions
- Reduce my stress so I can be more calm and focused on stage
- Build confidence to participate in a dance competition next year

Long-term goals typically have a time frame of around 1-5 years or more.

They should reflect your ultimate dance dreams, like dancing professionally, securing a college scholarship, or rising from the corps de ballet to soloist or principal.

Hint: Ensure you do not fall into the trap of comparing the time you need to accomplish a certain goal with someone else's timeline. Always remember that different dancers have different bodies and needs.

How to Stay Persistent with Your Goals

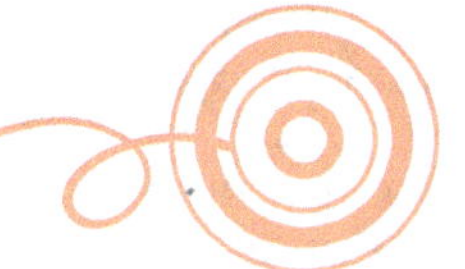

Be Mindful

Be mindful of creating goals that are too focused on something that is completely out of your control. For instance, it's not practical to say you want to be a principal dancer in a specific company, as ultimately, this decision lies with someone else. Instead, create goals that feed your confidence and improve you as a dancer, and then be open to the opportunities that come your way.

Also, setting too many goals at once can lead to frustration and anxiety, causing you to give up entirely. If you are a mid-level student, for example, you shouldn't try to work on as many goals as a professional dancer. Instead, create an effective plan using the S.M.A.R.T strategy and then diligently work on achieving one goal at time.

Check In

Every 3-4 weeks, remember to pause for a moment and check in with your goal. What have you achieved since you started working towards this goal? Aim to do this every 3-4 weeks. Be honest with yourself, and be reasonable. After all, ballet is a very demanding art and needs hard work and persistence. It is almost impossible to see noticeable improvement in just a few days' time, and by reviewing your progress too soon, it is easy to get frustrated. However, if you don't see improvement after a month or so of honest work, consider how else you might approach your goal. For example, you might consider asking a teacher for specific advice.

Focus on the Progress

When reviewing your progress, try not to fixate on whether or not you fully reached a goal, but rather on what you did achieve. This way, if you don't reach a goal but make a 50-percent improvement on where you were before, you will view it as a success. This will encourage you to keep pursuing the goal until you achieve it completely.

Adjust Where Necessary

Done right, goal setting is a continuous process. Whenever you achieve a goal, set another that aims to take you higher or focuses on a different area.

This way, you will persistently encourage yourself to improve. Review your goals frequently, and adjust them where necessary.

For example, if a goal turns out to be overly challenging and unachievable, alter it to something more suited to your current skill level.

Enjoy the Process

Goals will vary from person to person. It's important that you remain motivated and devoted to making your dream a reality by setting your own goals and then working to make them a reality.

In order to stay persistent and not give up, it is important that you exercise grit, patience, positivity and a hopeful attitude. A great tool is to concentrate on and visualize the end result. As a ballet dancer, you can stay persistent by setting a pragmatic schedule, allocating specific time each day to work on achieving your goal, and surrounding yourself with people who are also positive and working on their own goals. Practice self-care to re-energize yourself and ensure you keep giving your best – and don't forget to enjoy the process!

Set Your Own Goals

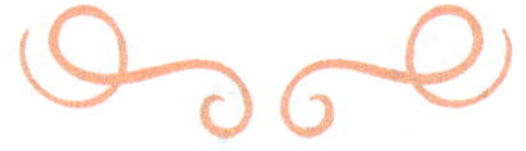

Studies suggest that you are 50% more likely to obtain your goals if you commit them to writing. The tone in which you write your goals should be resolute and unshakeable. The goals themselves should be realistic and attainable, yet challenging enough to help you grow. The best way to do this is to separate your goals to outcome goals and process goals.

Outcome goals cover what you want to achieve; they are the image you have in your mind that will make you excited and fulfilled when you will achieve it.

Process goals are the daily habits and actions you need to take that with consistency and repetition will lead you to reach your outcome goals. You should first check your lifestyle goals, which will help you improve your mental goals, which will help you excel in your training goals!

For example:
My lifestyle goal is to sleep at least eight hours every night, which will make me hit my mental goal to have less stress and better clarity in my day. This will help me train more effectively, with more focus and positivity.

Those process goals then will help me achieve my outcome goal, which is to enter the competition at the end of the year. This will boost my confidence and help me reach my long-term goal of auditioning for a place in my favorite company.

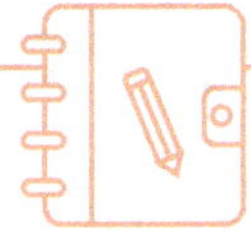
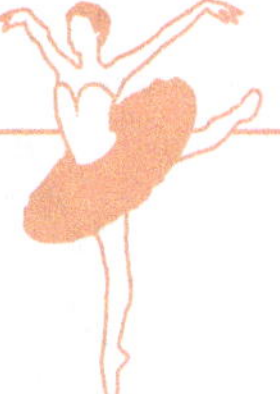

YOUR OUTCOME GOALS

Put your dream on paper. Make it specific. What do you truly want to achieve? Write down your "I want" statements.

Long-term Goals (1 - 5 years)

Short-term Goals (3 - 12 months)

YOUR PROCESS GOALS

Write down your habits and actions that will help you achieve the above goals:

Lifestyle Goals	Training Goals	Mental Goals

Manifest Your Goals

Visualize your goals achieved, a reality you've manifested. Feel the immense satisfaction and pride radiating from within, a warmth that fills every fiber of your being.

Write about your outcome goals as if they were already happening in your life. Describe in detail and present tense how happy and grateful you are.

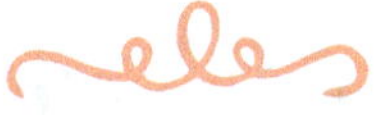

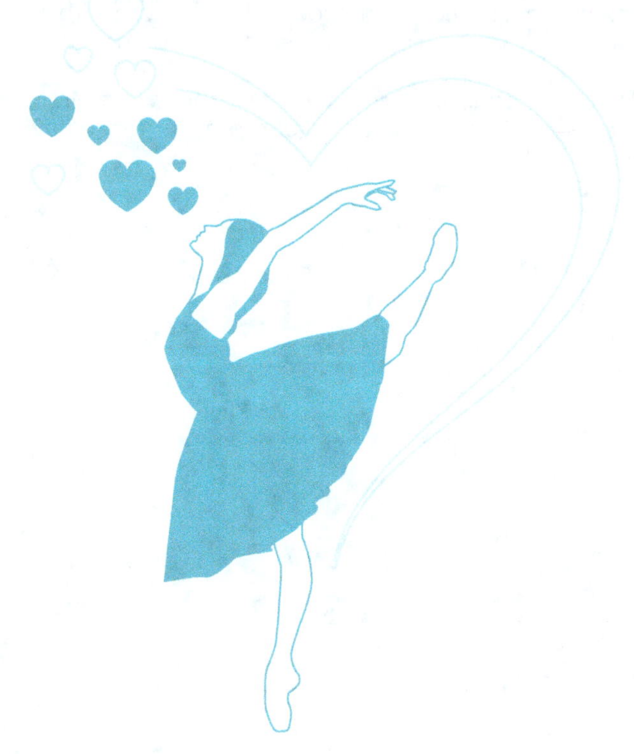

Positive Self-Talk

Craft your Inner Voice into your most Powerful Ally

"Words matter. And the words that matter most are the ones you say to yourself."

David Taylor-Klaus

Take a moment to think about how often you find yourself criticizing the way you look or perform.

At times, this little voice in our head can be positive and useful for keeping us motivated. But taking into consideration the focus, determination and perfectionist qualities that ballet dancers usually lean toward, we often become very critical of our dancing, and the way we see ourselves in class or on stage.

Audition didn't go your way? Does it fuel self-doubt, or does it spark a fire to work even harder for the next opportunity?

New choreography learned? Does it spark excitement or overwhelm you with self-doubt?

Misstep during the finale? Does your inner voice focus on the stumble, or does it celebrate the overall performance and your dedication?

How do you talk to yourself in the above situations? Is your inner voice helping, or could it be hurting? What kind of words do you usually use in these situations?

Let's pause and evaluate exactly what you're saying to yourself, as self-talk can be your greatest strength or your biggest enemy.

Dancers often don't realize how much they are holding themselves back by dancing from a place of self-judgment and doubt. Negative self-talk leads to anger, frustration, jealousy and restlessness, which challenges breathing, increases muscle tension, and affects concentration and focus. And all of this results in poorer performance and dramatically less joy while dancing.

Negative self-talk can increase self-doubt by limiting your potential, thinking and your ability to achieve your goals and dreams. Every time you repeat negative words to yourself you are reinforcing and strengthening their message in your mind, making it a part of your belief system.

A belief is something we consider to be a fact. It is anything we assume to be true. We all have our own set of them, called our belief system. Our belief system is powerful and affects almost everything we think, feel and do. It influences our emotions and actions. Our beliefs also dictate what we consider possible or achievable. You may have already heard the saying "believing is achieving." Understand that a particular belief can limit or enhance your performance.

Your linguistic memory consists of words and phrases that you use repeatedly. Thanks to the power that repetition – along with your deep faith in them – gives these phrases, they will become your reality. If these words and phrases are negative, they will cause you to become upset instead of calm, frustration instead of motivation and will eventually become a bad habit… and bad habits steal a lot from our best selves.

Words such as "cannot," "will not," "could have," and "should have," indicate a lack of self-belief. They have been shown to increase both somatic (physical) and cognitive anxiety.

The more you tell yourself that you can't perform well, the more your brain will start believing and acting that way, depriving you of new experiences and opportunities to learn and grow. The words you use when speaking to yourself have the potential to make or break you. Using them wisely is crucial.

To sum up, negative self-talk:

- Affects your enjoyment of dance

- Shatters your confidence

- Makes you feel depressed, anxious, and lost

- Pulls you downward rather than lifting up your performance

- Sends the message to yourself that you are not good enough, and that no matter what you accomplish, it's not good enough either

- Increases muscle tension and creates a loss of concentration and focus.

We often don't even realize that we are behaving like our own worst enemy by letting such destructive and negative words and thoughts breed in our mind.
In ballet, intense competition and perfectionism can create a lot of self-talk, so it is really important that you become your own biggest supporter. You must be able to withstand the criticism that will come your way by creating an internal layer of positive self-talk.

Even if your mind is engulfed by negative thoughts and patterns, you can break free from it by monitoring your thoughts closely. With consistency and daily practice, you can develop a new belief system that is much more powerful, encouraging, uplifting and motivating.

By adopting positive self-talk, you can totally transform the way you feel about yourself and become the best dancer you can be. So let's see how you can use positive self-talk to your own advantage.

Positive Self-Talk

When you exercise positive self-talk, you create an optimistic state of mind that helps you manage everyday stress in a more constructive way. That ability may contribute to the widely observed health benefits of positive thinking, including increased life span, better cardiovascular health and lower rates of depression.

Neuroscientist Andrew Newberg and communications expert Mark Robert Waldman explain that when the parietal and frontal lobes of the brain are stimulated with a positive word or thought, a message is sent from the chamber to other parts of the brain, which blocks the ability of the limbic system to produce neurochemical signals that cause distress, irritability and anger.

So positive self-talk gives you a dose of energy, strength, and good vibes. It's a blend of courage and stamina that allows you to take new leaps in life. Positive self-talk is promising and alluring, reassuring you that "you can do this," "you can make it," "you are enough." It allows you to believe you can achieve your goals and dreams, despite any obstacles or difficulties that may occur.

 Positive self-talk isn't about thinking you're flawless or surpassing emotions like anger, sadness or fear; it's simply about changing the way you look at things – removing negative bias, and developing the belief that you can face and overcome your challenges. Positive self-talk looks like this: "I feel really sad that I wasn't chosen to dance this role, but I am strong, confident and persistent so I am sure I will make it next time."

Positive self-talk is not about avoiding difficult situations, it is about altering the way you approach stressful situations, and approaching challenges to the best of your ability. It's about knowing that whatever the outcome, you did the best you could, and will learn from your mistakes for next time.

So let's see how you can improve your self-talk.

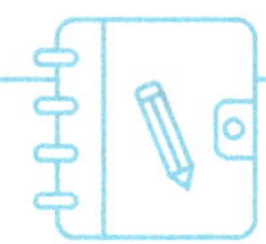

NOTING

In this exercise we will use a technique called Noting. It will help you expand your awareness of your self-talk's quality.

For the next week, whenever you catch yourself self-talking, try to put a mental note on that self-talk. Whether you are practicing, rehearsing or watching someone else perform, if your mind wanders, try to bring it back to awareness and put a label to the words or phrases you use while you self-talk. It is important that you don't judge or become critical of your thoughts; just add a mental note to them like an objective observer: Are they positive or negative?

Some examples are:

- I can't do this!
- I'm not good enough.
- Oh! Why is my turnout so terrible?
- I'm gonna mess up this part of the choreography again.
- Everyone is a better turner than me.
- I'm very proud of my progress.
- I have a great sense of musicality.
- Great try!

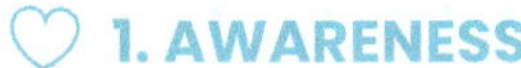

♡ 1. AWARENESS

Write down those words or phrases

POSITIVE   NEGATIVE

☆ 2. EVALUATION

a. Ask yourself the following questions:

Am I using mostly positive or negative words and phrases?

What usually triggers these thoughts?

- Criticism from teachers

- Comparison with other dancers

b. Write down the three negative words and phrases that you use the most:

NEGATIVE

c. Ask yourself

- How do these words or statements make me feel?

3. LIBERATION

"Rephrasing negative statements into positive and empowering ones can be a great tool that will change the overall quality of your dance life."For example, if you wrote on the negative list: "I'm not gonna make it," you can rephrase it with:

Even if it's difficult, I can do it.
If I try hard, I'll get there!
I know it's super demanding but with discipline and hard work, I can make it happen!
I've overcome so many challenges! That is what I'm gonna do again.

Notice in the above examples that you start to change the phrase to positive while keeping mention of the difficult part. Do not just start using positive statements. The point of this exercise is not to fool yourself or underestimate the difficulty you are facing, but to reframe the challenge in a positive way. We want to be realistic without resorting to bad self-criticism.

REPHRASING

....

....

....

....

....

Finally, take a moment to notice what happens to your temper, your psychology and your body when you replace the negative statements with positive ones.

Hint: Don't forget that our mind tends to fall back to its old habits, so it is important to go back to this exercise often. It is like building muscle or learning a new skill. The more you do it, the stronger you get. With time and practice you will be able to "catch" negative statements the moment they arise and turn them into useful and productive ones.

SELF-TALK TIPS FOR DANCERS

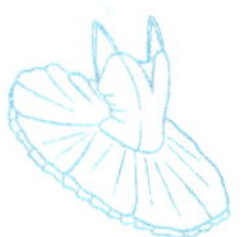

Ballet life throws curveballs – challenges, breakthroughs, and yes, exhaustion! But that's when positive self-talk becomes your secret weapon, fueling your resilience.

I can do it... I know I'm capable of... It is possible to succeed... Let's try this again... Let's go strong... Keep it up... Stay focused... Good job... Setback today, stronger tomorrow... One step at a time, I'll get there... I'll enjoy practicing... Despite feeling worn out and stressed, I gave it my all...

These are some phrases you can utilize before, during, and after a class, rehearsal, or performance. They can provide the uplift, bravery, and positivity you might need to tackle these demanding situations. Many of these statements reinforce the idea that you have the necessary skills, positive mindset, and convictions for a successful performance.

Your Positive Self-Talk Collection

Write down your own words and phrases that serve the above purposes so you can have them available in class.

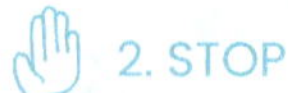 ## 2. STOP

The moment you realize you are using words like "can't," "won't," "will never," " I never," say "Stop!" either aloud or to yourself.

Take three deep breaths and notice the negative self-talk. Don't criticize yourself about it, and don't try to immediately push it away. Just notice it for a bit.

Then replace the phrase with a positive one from your collection.

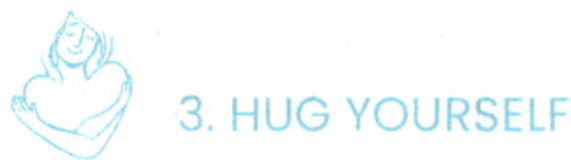 ## 3. HUG YOURSELF

Dance days can be tough, and the inner critic can get downright loud sometimes. But before you get caught in that negativity spiral, hit pause and ask yourself:

Would you ever rip into your best friend with harsh words after a setback? Of course not! You'd offer support and encouragement, reminding them of their strengths.

Show yourself the same compassion you'd show a friend. Replace the self-doubt with gentle affirmations and celebrate your wins, big and small. Building a positive inner dialogue is like building a strong foundation for your dance journey. So, fill your self-talk with love and encouragement!

Don't forget to frequently embrace yourself.

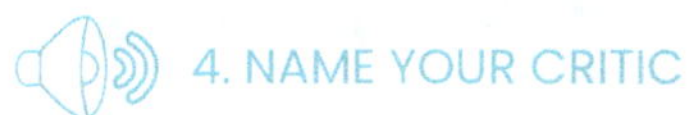

"Don't believe everything you tell yourself."
Lidia Longorio

An interesting and funny way to make our hypercritical inner voice lose its power is to give him or her a funny personality. Close your eyes and recall a moment when your critical voice appeared.

Now try to play a bit with your inner critic. Give it a funny look, a funny name, and most of all a funny voice. Imagine your inner voice sounding like Mickey Mouse or Spongebob, or someone equally as humorous. You could also imagine that it has a very funny appearance.

This will cause your critical inner voice
to lose some of its power, and it will become
easier to handle.

I mean, try to imagine Spongbob telling you, "You are worthless and you won't be able to make it!" You can't take that seriously and believe it, right?

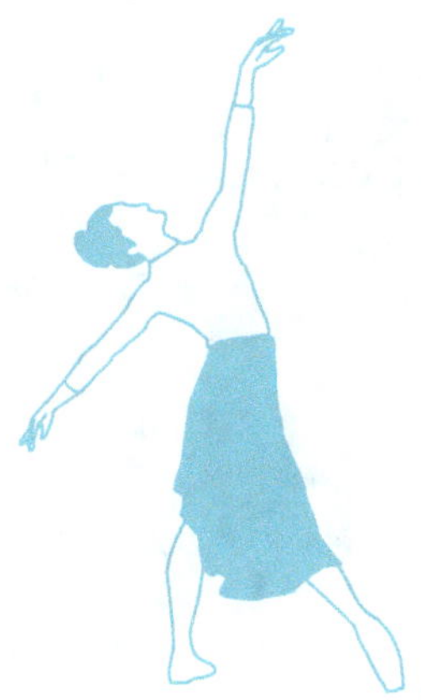

> *"You are the average of the five people you surround yourself with."*
> **Jim Rohn**

If there are negative, toxic or ungrateful people in your life, then you add all these qualities to your life as well.

We usually choose to surround ourselves with people who share common interests and goals. Ballet dancers usually choose other ballet dancers to hang out with after class, and that is normal.

But in the ballet field, where perfectionism and competitiveness are very common traits, dancers can easily feel unsatisfied and be very strict with themselves. And they usually carry this state back home or to their other social activities.

So be very careful with the people you choose to surround yourself with after class or in your social activities. Try to include people in your life that enrich you with positive qualities not solely related to ballet. Spend your time with people that are positive, optimistic, ambitious, fun and have a sense of humor.

You need to maintain a strong and positive mindset, devotion, passion and drive, and the people you surround yourself with will play an important role in that.

So, surround yourself with positive people in order to add more happiness and beautiful energy to your life!

Saying positive things about yourself each day will not only stop the chain of negative self-talk but will help you feel much better about yourself in general. The following affirmations are powerful tools you can use anywhere, anytime – in the studio, out of the studio, and even during rehearsals. It will help you push through your toughest days and motivate you to always give your best.

Use some of the affirmations below or create your own:

- I am confident, strong and beautiful.
- I have all the capabilities to succeed in ballet.
- My love for ballet cannot be diminished by any sort of criticism.
- Ballet dancing is my passion.
- I love myself the way I am.
- Today is going to be a great day.
- I am strong enough to face any challenge.
- A bad day in class or rehearsal doesn't affect me.
- I will support myself no matter what.
- Mistakes and failures don't define me.
- I learn from my mistakes and will come back even stronger than before.
- I am very focused on giving my best performance.
- I am proud of how far I have come.

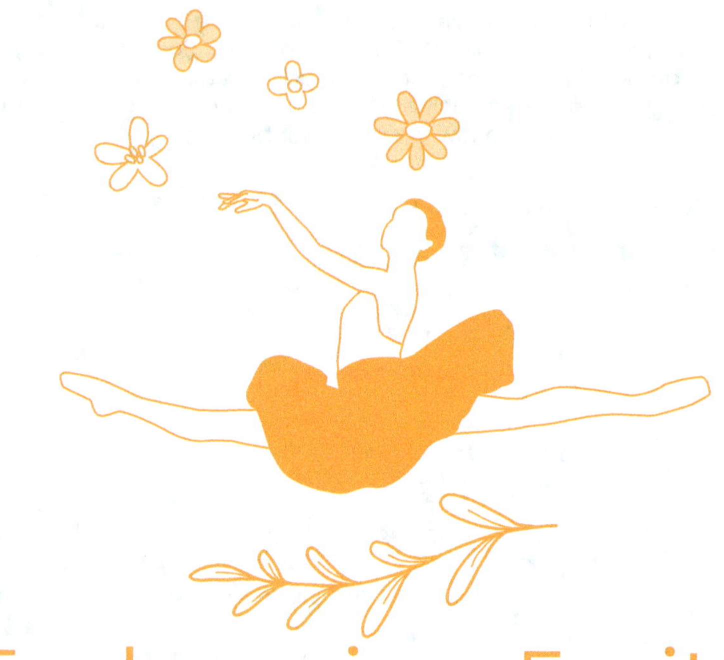

Embracing Fruitful Failure

Turn setbacks into stepping stones for unstoppable success

"As young creative artists, and really as human beings, you have to be open to failure. Failure is a part of learning.

...As a very old dancer, I have had many, many opportunities to fail. It happens. Projects collapse, knees blow out, money dries up. But you as artists, and as young people discovering what you care about, you must be generous to that spark inside yourself that made you love dance in the first place."

Mikhail Baryshnikov

Dancers work really hard and devote themselves to their art, and a "failure" in a competition, audition, performance, or even in class, can threaten their sense of self or dancing skills.

Failure usually causes pain. And pain, whether emotional or physical, is something we naturally try to avoid at all costs. Many times we try to avoid failure by not accepting challenges, trying new things, or taking risks. This is because we can't stand the heavy emotion of not succeeding, and the negative criticism we believe will come from our peers, parents, teachers or directors.

Dancers who experience extreme concerns about mistakes, a more negative form of perfectionism, are particularly likely to feel shame or embarrassment after failure.

But despite all these uncomfortable emotions that "failure" causes us, failure is an essential component for our personal growth as ballet dancers. Failure is part of our success. And as dancers, we learn this from an early age, as we have to fail several times in order to see even a little progress in our technique.

We usually talk about the successes of the great dancers, but what we tend to forget is that they too failed many times before they succeeded – and they still "fail" sometimes.

A more constructive definition of failure is when an individual hasn't accomplished their intended goal – just YET.

Failure does not mean that we ourselves are failures; instead it means we are strong enough to face that failure, and that's why we were challenged by choosing to become dancers. Failure is an opportunity to learn from our mistakes and grow. It is a small setback that sets us up for something better and bigger. With time, failure brings us more maturity and experience.

Now that we know that failure is necessary for achieving our ballet dreams, let's see the bright side of it and make failure our greatest friend...

Let's embrace fruitful failure.

Benefits of Fruitful Failure

Failure comes with a lot of benefits, which is why we call it "fruitful failure." Here are some of the benefits you will experience even if you fail after giving your best in ballet dancing.

You Grow Positively

Failures and mistakes provide you with a valuable source of feedback. You recognize your limitations and how to work around them. Analyzing a bad day in class, performance, or an unsuccessful audition, helps you identify what you need to work on and where your weak areas are. Maybe you struggle with a technical step, or experience anxiety on stage. In this way, failures and mistakes highlight your weaknesses.

What's so wonderful about that, you may ask? Simple! It helps you get better, stronger, more confident and more skilled as a dancer. Knowing your weaknesses is crucial as it helps you analyze what didn't work in any given situation and identify areas for improvement and strategize on how to overcome them. Failure is useful feedback for what you need to do next time in order to grow as a dancer and be successful.

You Value Hard Work

Ballet isn't easy. You have to stay committed to hard work and continue improving your skills on a daily basis in order to achieve your goals. Remind yourself that success is based on steady, persistent discipline and hard work. Failure teaches you humility and gives you an appreciation of what it takes to be a successful dancer.

You Build Resilience

Failure strengthens our character, our commitment and our work ethics. The more often you successfully navigate failure, the stronger and more resilient you become. When you physically fall and must pick yourself back up, you build muscle and strength. Similarly, each time you fail and bounce back, you build confidence and self-esteem.

You Learn That It's Not Always About You

After not being accepted by the dance company you have always wanted to join, or not getting your dream role, it can feel like the world has ended. But your failures often involve many factors beyond your control.

For example, there are many reasons why you might not have gotten a contract. The director may have been looking for a certain height or body type, for instance. Instead of dwelling on things you can't change, do your best to stay positive, grow more as a dancer and focus on your goals..

It Will Make Your Success Worth It

Succeeding after repeated failure is one of the greatest feelings in the world. No matter how challenging it can be to get back on track after failing, not giving up will only be in your favor for the future. When you finally live your dream, great satisfaction and pride will fill every inch of you, knowing that all the failure, rejections and criticism you went through were totally worth it.

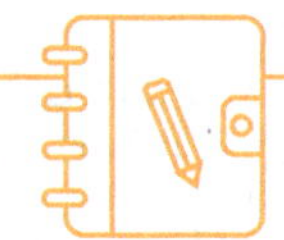

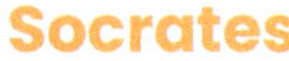

Fruitful Failure Tools

"Falling down is not a failure. Failure comes when you stay where you have fallen."

Socrates

Turning Failure Into Fruitful Failure

After a failure, it can be all too easy to criticize ourselves and focus on the negative. Instead, a great approach after a struggle is to ask yourself these four questions:

1. What went well?

2. What could have been done differently?

3. What needs work?

4. What can I learn from today that will help me perform better in the future?

It is really important to add the element of positivity into the evaluation of each failure. This way, we learn to see some good in the bad and also spot the opportunities that may arise.

Fruitful Failure Reminder 

After a failure, always remind yourself:

→ Mistakes and failures are part of the path to achieving my goals.

→ Failures give me an opportunity to learn and become a better dancer.

→ I will not allow myself to remain stuck in frustration.

→ I will stay positive and continue to strive for the best possible result.

Share Your Failures 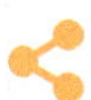

After a failure, feelings like disappointment, anger and frustration usually arise. Remember that there's no shame in being frustrated or disappointed. Allow yourself to express your feelings and share your feelings with a good friend.

But never let the difficult feelings keep you from returning to the studio the next day with the discipline, perspective, faith and open mind that will make you the best dancer you can be.

Remember, what you may consider a failure right now is merely a stepping stone to get you where you want and need to be.

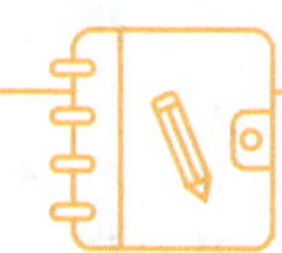

Embracing the Stumble

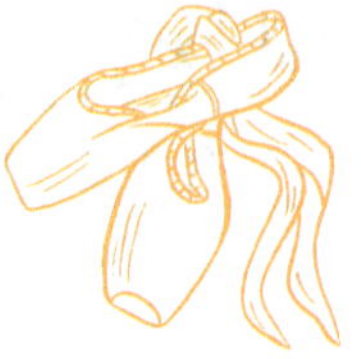

This exercise will help you transform failure into
a valuable ally on your ballet journey.

Part 1: Reflecting on a Fall

1. Recall a recent experience in ballet where you felt you "failed." This
could be anything from a missed step in class to a disappointing
performance.

2. Describe the situation in detail. What were you trying to achieve?
What happened?

3. Identify the emotions you felt. Did you feel embarrassed, frustrated, or discouraged?

4. Analyze the cause of the "failure." Was it a technical issue, a mental block, or something else entirely?

5. Write down at least two possible lessons you can learn from this
experience. For example, did you need to practice a specific step
more, or would visualization exercises help you stay focused during
performances?

Part 2: Reframing the Fall

1. Rewrite the narrative of your "failure." Instead of focusing on the negative emotions, see this as an opportunity for growth.

2. Imagine a famous ballet dancer facing a similar setback. How might they react? What advice would they offer you?

3. Turn your lessons learned into a confidence booster. For example, "Even the most graceful dancers stumble sometimes," or "Mistakes are stepping stones to improvement."

4. Visualize yourself successfully overcoming this "failure" in the future. See yourself executing the step flawlessly, or delivering a captivating performance.

5. Write a positive affirmation for yourself. "I am a resilient dancer who learns from my mistakes," or "I embrace challenges and celebrate progress."

Remember, every great dancer has stumbled in the studio. By embracing these stumbles as learning experiences, you can turn failure into your greatest ally and propel yourself towards achieving your ballet dreams.

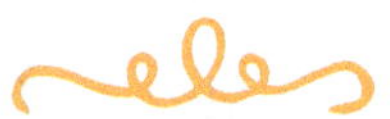

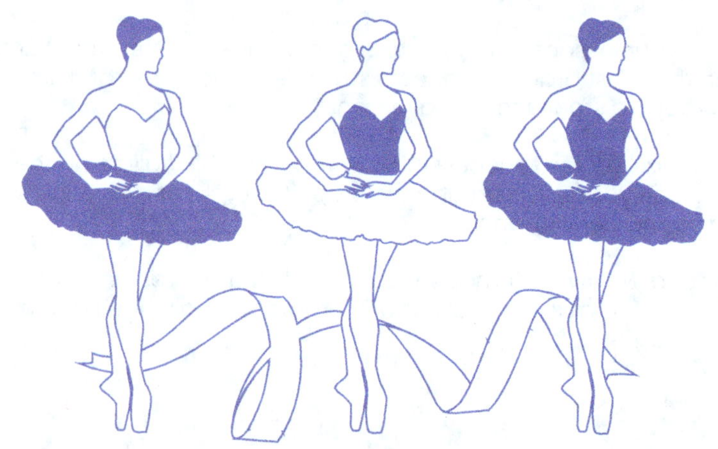

The Comparison Trap

Find Inspiration and Unleash Your Artistic Brilliance

Of course you have.

All dancers experience times when they feel challenged or that they are be-ing left behind, and as a result, they start comparing themselves to others. This is very much expected because you are continuously watching and analyzing your fellow dancers, not just in class but on the stage, on social media, even in changing rooms. There will always be someone with higher extensions, more turnout, and maybe stronger technique than you do.

Dancers shine in their own unique way. One dancer may be a great turn-er, while another may be an excellent jumper. One dancer may dance in a tense, energetic way, while another in a softer and more fluid way. One dancer may be incredibly expressive, while another concentrates more on technique.

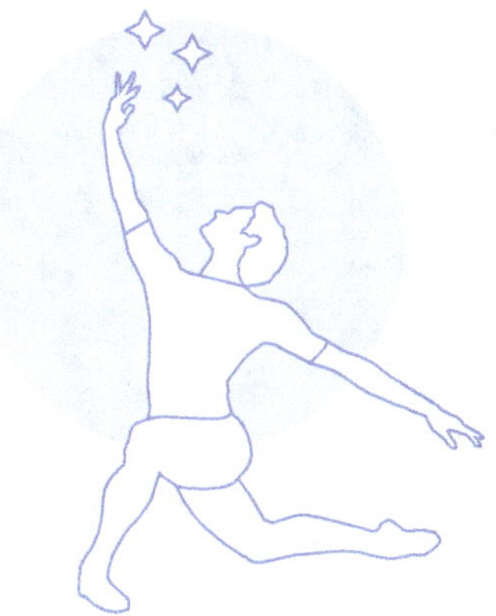

One thing is for sure: all dancers are different. Different qualities, strengths and weaknesses; and all without ex-ception need to strive for something.

So you must always keep in mind your uniqueness. Your special features that differentiate you from other dancers.

And don't forget that ballet is not only about the physical characteristics. A focused and positive mindset is more important than anything else. A focused mindset will keep you aligned with your goals, whatever the difficul-ties and drawbacks. It will help you approach each struggle from a healthy perspective and keep you from making reactive, destructive decisions.

There are very good dancers who suffer due to a lack of mental features like confidence, motivation, stress management skills, and healthy habits. The bottom line is that every dancer has struggles. While you might be having difficulties improving your jumps and boosting your confidence, another person could be grappling with issues in refining their turns and maintaining proper nutrition. Similarly, a different individual might be dealing with an entirely different set of struggles.But whatever we say about how unproductive and useless it is to compare ourselves to others, it is almost impossible to not do it.

So let's discover a wiser and more productive way to do so!

The Circle of Negative Comparison

"When you continuously compete with others, you become bitter. But when you continuously compete with yourself, you become better."

Marie Blanchard

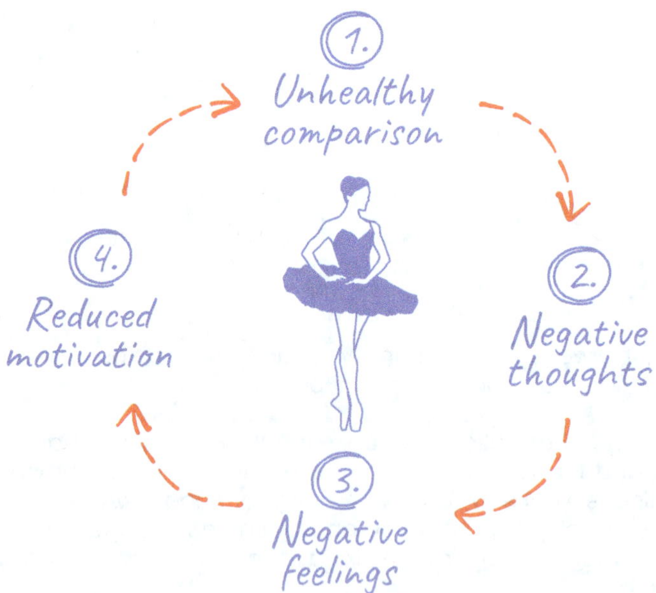

There is no winner in negative comparison. As you can see, negative comparison almost always leads to negative thoughts.

"They have nicer lines, a better body, stronger technique," etc.

And the more you focus on them, the more these negative thoughts increase!

These thoughts then lead to negative emotions such as frustration, anger, jealousy and feelings of injustice.

"Why them and not me?"

This is the moment we may begin to feel inferior. Then, our sense of self-worth begins to blur and motivation reduces or gets completely lost. Along with generating negative thoughts and feelings within us, this comparison also distracts us from our goals.

The energy we could have invested in chasing our dreams is wasted on feeling frustrated and maybe jealous of other people's success and strengths. This prevents us from making any sort of progress and discovering our own value and potential.

We also steal from ourselves precious moments of joy, pride and fulfillment that we could have experienced after achieving different goals. By focusing on what other dancers have that you don't, you are giving your time, energy and power away. Every second you spend comparing your path to someone else's could be used to create and achieve your own goals.

The Circle of Productive Comparison

The Circle of Productive Comparison works in the exact opposite way:

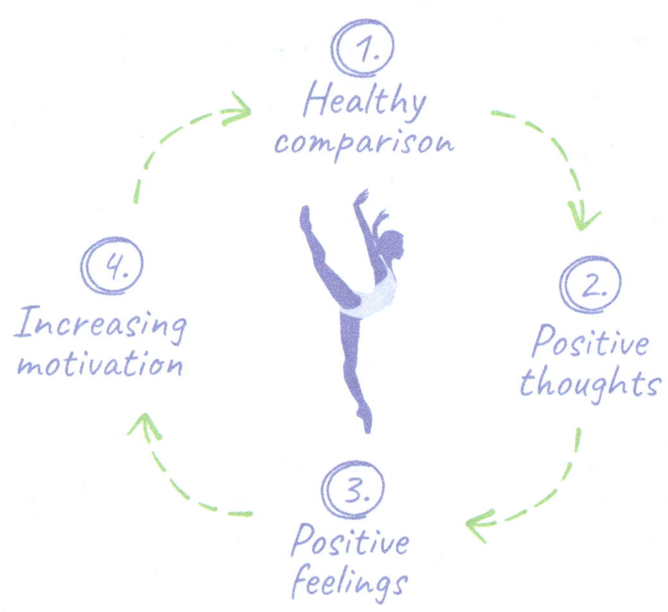

What you need to do in order to experience its beautiful benefits is to make a mental shift... and let other dancers inspire you!

Move from a self-evaluation comparison – which happens when a person is trying to compare their own attributes, skills and capabilities with others – to a self-improvement comparison, which allows people to get inspired by others' skills. Through this method of comparison, you are able to observe people in order to improve your own skills and learn to deal with problems in a better way.

Take a minute to observe and admire every single beautiful feature they have. Maybe it is the way they work, their beautiful legs, their precise technique, their musicality, how determined they are to succeed, their tenacity, passion or persistence.

In the beginning, it's not easy to feel that way; this is normal, given how competitive the ballet field is. How can you feel this way about dancers who are potential "rivals?" That could take your place in a company? Or could they get a role you've always wanted?"

But that is the great shift you need to make. Use our tendency to compare ourselves, but do it in a positive and helpful way.

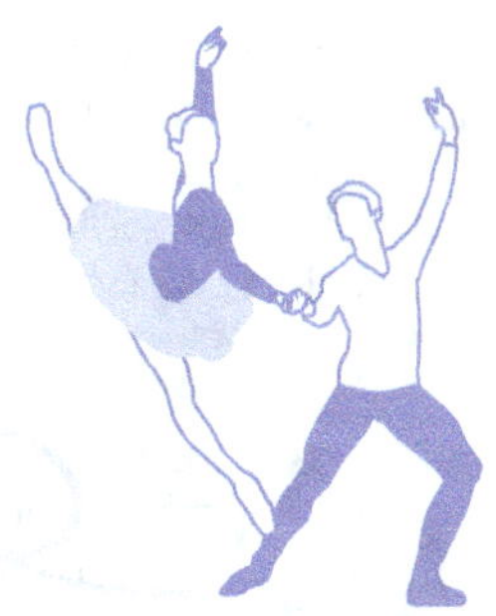

This approach will always create positive emotions. It will motivate you, give you a great boost, and increase your passion to achieve even more. That way, you create happiness instead of disappointment, jealousy and negativity.

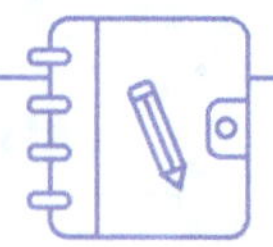

Tips for Avoiding the Comparison Trap

1. Focus on Yourself and Be Mindful of Your Own Thoughts

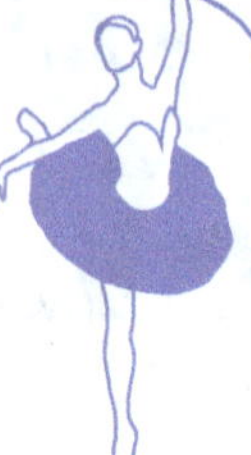

> "I do not try to dance better than anyone else, I only try to dance better than myself."
>
> **Mikhail Baryshnikov**

The brain is a muscle that can be trained according to what we feed it with. So it's very important to be mindful of your thoughts.

The more you change your thoughts, beliefs and intentions behind comparison, the sooner your mind will be trained to think differently about it.

Every time you find yourself making comparisons with others, try to stop yourself, take a deep breath and switch your focus towards something productive, positive and inspiring. It's easier said than done, but with persistence it is possible.

Here is a list of actions you can take in order to focus all your attention and energy on yourself when you fall into the comparison trap:

- Go back to your Goal Setting Tool and re-read your goals. That way you turn your focus to the things you are striving for.

- Practice a 10-minute mindfulness meditation so you can be aware of your thoughts and get back to your center.

- Consume inspiring content like interviews from your favorite dancers or listen to dance podcasts.

- Book your next Pilates or yoga class.

- Celebrate your progress! Feel happy, proud and fulfilled for every little milestone you achieve!

- Remind yourself that there are so many things to do for yourself and your dream! Put all your energy there. There's no time to waste on petty comparisons!

2. Use Social Media Wisely 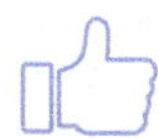

You know very well that competition within a school or company is stressful enough as we're forced to dance side by side in front of a mirror. On top of that, nowadays we can compare ourselves not only to our peers in class but to dancers from all over the world through social media. There's no easier way to get down on yourself if you don't use social media wisely.

It is really easy to fall into the comparison trap when we're confronted with all those "perfect" images, which most of the time are far from reality. You may see amazing poses but you don't know anything about these dancers. An out-of-this-world pose on its own doesn't mean anything.

If you really want to find inspiration through social media, look for signs of real training and artistic quality in dancers' profiles.

A great way to use social media wisely is: 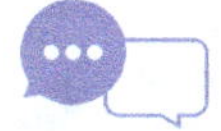

- Ask yourself a daily question: Have I triggered my Negative or my Productive Comparison Circle after using social media?

- Use the Inspire or Unfollow rule: If the account you follow inspires, motivates and makes you feel good about yourself, continue to follow it. If not, it's better to unfollow it even for a while (give a try) just to notice how you feel. I'm sure you won't regret it!

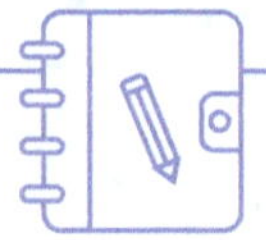

EXERCISES FOR BOOSTING YOUR PRODUCTIVE COMPARISON CIRCLE

Gratitude

There is nothing more beautiful and powerful than being able to recognize and feel grateful for your own strengths and talents. Identify and write down what is unique about you. Remind yourself of your strengths! Your true potential! Your true worth!

Write down all your physical and mental strengths and your deep personal values in order to have an overall picture of who you are. Every time you fall into the comparison trap, redirect your focus to this list, reminding yourself of your true value.

Physical Strengths	Mental Strengths	Personal Values
1	1	1 ....
2	2	2 ....
3	3	3 ....

Trigger Awareness

This week, try to watch yourself, and every time you catch yourself making comparisons to others, make a note in your journal or your mind. Later, in a quiet space, answer the following questions:

- What traits in others do I frequently compare myself to? (body appearance, extensions, confidence)

....

- Why am I comparing these specific things about myself to others? (What kind of insecurity wakes me up and makes me worry?)

....

- How does this comparison make me feel?
  (less capable, worthless, bad)

....

- How much time did I spend in that negative state of mind?

....

Focus on Self-discovery

Comparing always stems from some kind of insecurity or fear and a deeper search may be necessary to find the root cause.

Work on learning more about yourself and your patterns either through mindfulness, therapy or any other self-awareness method. It is one of the best investments you can make in yourself, as it will allow you to take conscious control of your life and your choices.

Your self-discovery trip should include:

✔ Uncovering your insecurities and identifying their trigger points.

✔ Learning to be kind to your insecurities rather than judgmental. Learn to show love and empathy toward them.

✔ Learning how to share your issues with a good friend, in order to understand and realize that you're not the only person with insecurities! Insecurity and fear is a shared human feature.

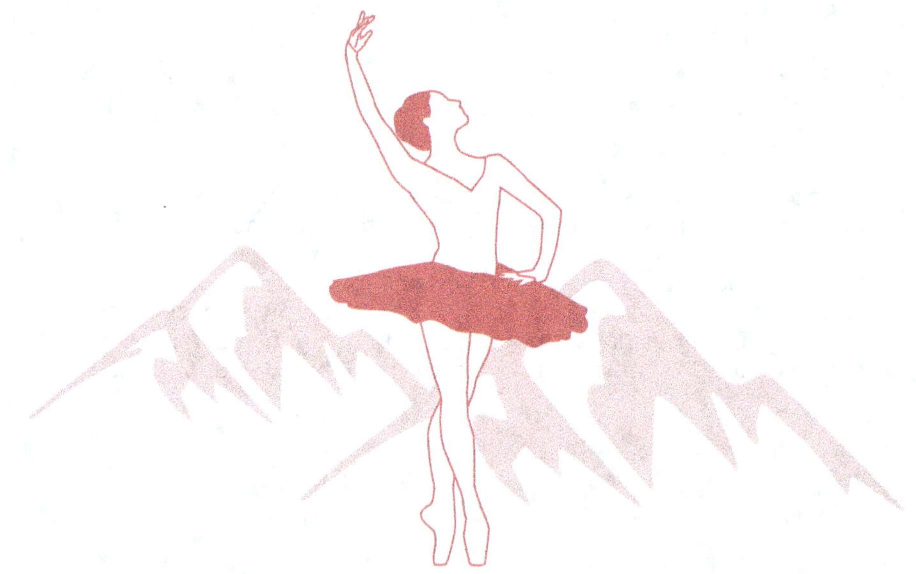

Turn Up
the Confidence

Believe in the Power Within You

"If you want to live your ballet dream, you will have to work consistently and persistently on your confidence". Years of experience highlight its crucial role in achieving success.

Confidence is a belief that you can perform at your best and reach your goals. It's a strong faith in yourself and your strengths. It's the certainty that you can succeed.

Think about what usually holds you back from having constant confidence in your dance. Is it:

- The criticism/corrections that you get from your teachers or choreographers?

- The comparisons you make between yourself and other dancers?

- The voice inside your head telling you that you are not good enough?

- Past bad experiences that you keep repeating in your head?

The list can be never-ending!

But it is important to know that confidence is a skill that can be developed through practice and experience – and all of us can build it.

So, whatever it is that may break your confidence – your thoughts, your past failures or the world around you – you have to take charge of building, sustaining and protecting your confidence.

Inviting confidence into your life will not only make you more focused on your goals but will also help your personality shine.

So let's take a look at how you can work on building lasting confidence that can assist you in becoming a great ballet dancer!

The Three Types of Confidence

The following are the three major types of confidence:

1. Under-confidence can be explained as a low level of confidence and poor self-esteem that prevents you from seeing your real potential as a dancer. Oftentimes, it can result in feelings of insecurity, self-doubt and worthlessness. If you have low confidence, it's easy to get intimidated and influenced by other people. You are oversensitive to criticism and may feel very anxious when you have to perform due to fear of other people's judgments about your mistakes or performance. This fear makes you avoid stepping out of your comfort zone and thus hinders your growth.

2. Self-confidence is the trust you have in your own abilities. It is the awareness of your own strengths and limitations and the ability to use these to your advantage. It encourages you to seek out challenging choreography and varied career opportunities. You are not scared of failure; instead you use challenging experiences to learn something new, or to perform even better next time. You are open to your teacher's or choreographer's suggestions and opinions, and welcome constructive feedback to assist in your growth. At the same time, you know how to deal with negative feedback. You have trust in your preparation and you are willing to take calculated risks and strike a healthy balance between too little and too much confidence about your own capabilities; as a result, your dancing improves.

3. Over-confidence can refer to excessive belief in your own abilities to the level where it is unrealistic. This can lead to narcissistic and egoistic behavior, which prevents you from listening to teachers' suggestions and feedback, thus hindering your growth. This often lands you in overwhelming and difficult situations, due to the overestimation of your own abilities and a propensity to take on high-risk challenges.

How to Increase Self-Confidence

Practice, Practice, Practice!

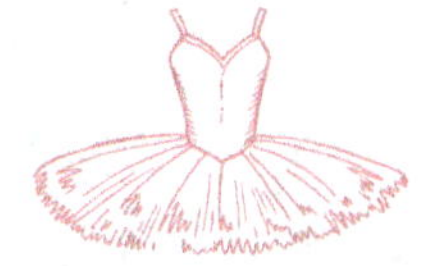

There is no substitute for hard work.

Confidence alone is not enough to make you succeed; you must also have the necessary ability. Self-confidence comes out of a solid base of physical and mental training. Your confidence increases together with the skills that you build through your hard work every day.

Set yourself goals and keep working hard to reach them. Work hard on your weaknesses and make them your main priority in your training. Challenge yourself and do whatever is necessary in order to improve. There is no greater satisfaction than seeing your weaknesses gradually turn into strengths. When progress and development come, your pride, satisfaction, and happiness will be enormous. There's no greater boost for your confidence.

If you want to be the best dancer you can be, remember, there's no room for complacency! Continue to develop your strengths so they have an even greater positive effect on your confidence and performances. Make them your best and brightest traits!

Give 100% of your effort each day and let the gradual progress increase your confidence. Remember that confidence comes from knowing you've trained smarter and harder than yesterday.

Challenge Yourself on a Daily Basis

In order to become more confident, it's important to overcome your fears. For that to happen, you need to have the courage to get out of your comfort zone and do things you usually hesitate to do.

For some, that may mean putting themselves in the front row of the class instead of hiding in the corner. For others, it means overcoming a fear of failure and making the decision to participate in a competition. Or it may mean striving for more pirouettes, fouettés and higher jumps!

Set your own challenges and find the courage and faith to overcome them. Challenge yourself to see what you can become. Remember that challenging roads always lead to beautiful destinations.

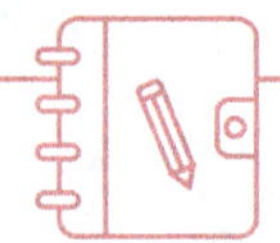

Self-Confidence Boost Exercise

This exercise will help you discover the factors that increase or decrease your confidence levels – and figure out a way to overcome them.

a. High Confidence

First write down the situations or qualities in your dance life that make you feel confident.

For example: "I learn new choreography quickly."

High Confidence List

1 . . . .

2 . . . .

3 . . . .

Now close your eyes and visualize yourself in these situations. Let yourself feel grateful for having these unique qualities that make you feel confident.

b. Low Confidence

Now write down the situations or qualities in your dance life that make you feel less confident. By putting these situations on paper and clearly identifying them, you become more aware of them.

For example: "When I transition from the dance studio to the stage, I find my confidence wavering due to the absence of a mirror for self-checking and rectification"

Low Confidence List

1 . . . .

2 . . . .

3 . . . .

Now write down what you can do in order to manage those low-confidence situations better. For example:

"A few days before I go on stage, I'll stop looking at myself in the mirror while dancing."

"I will reduce my stress and increase my concentration by doing mindfulness meditation before I go on stage."

"I will use visualization to improve my sense of control and stability in every movement."

"I will record myself in order to check that what I feel is real, and make all necessary corrections."

What can I do to manage the above Low Confidence list?

1 ....

....

2 ....

....

3 ....

....

Come back to this exercise often in order to reevaluate the situations that may break your confidence and plan your steps for dealing with them.

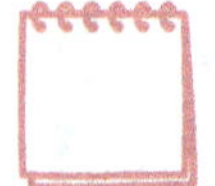

Self-Confidence Tips for Dancers

Acknowledge Your Little Daily Wins

You don't need to achieve the big things in life in order to build your confidence. Appreciate yourself for doing the right things every day. Small improvements happen every day whether it's within the dynamic environment of a classroom, amidst the creative energy of a rehearsal, or during a carefully structured pilates session.

If you train yourself to acknowledge your little daily wins you will have a continuous flow of positive emotions, excitement, pride and satisfaction. These are all great elements for building your confidence slowly but deeply every day, as you will be able to see and feel yourself improving your technique, your strength and your performance and getting closer to your goals.

Write your little wins in your journal each day, and take a moment to reflect on them. This can be a great daily confidence booster.

Stop Comparing Yourself to Others

As we already mentioned in this guide, comparison is one of the biggest confidence killers. It can really affect your performance and cause you to lose sight of your goals.

Go back to the Comparison Trap Tool in this guide and work on boosting your Productive Comparison Circle if you haven't done so already.

Manage Unrealistic Expectations

Try not to set the bar too high! Ensure your confidence is reasonable and that you don't set unrealistic expectations.

Additionally, avoid the pitfall of perfectionism that can perpetually leave you feeling inadequate or under-accomplished. Setting unrealistic standards or striving for perfection can blind you to the significant progress you've made through dedication and effort.

Later in this guide, you will find the Perfectionism Tool. This will help you work more deeply on that subject.

Use Positive Self-talk

Positive self-talk can change the way you feel and think about yourself and can ultimately affect your level of confidence.

At each and every point of your training, remind yourself how capable and deserving you are. Encourage and appreciate yourself at every little success. Along with increasing your confidence level, positive self-talk also makes your training more enjoyable and productive.

Go back to the Self-talk Tool if necessary to reevaluate the quality of your self-talk.

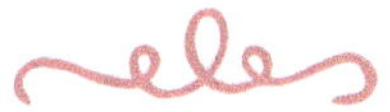

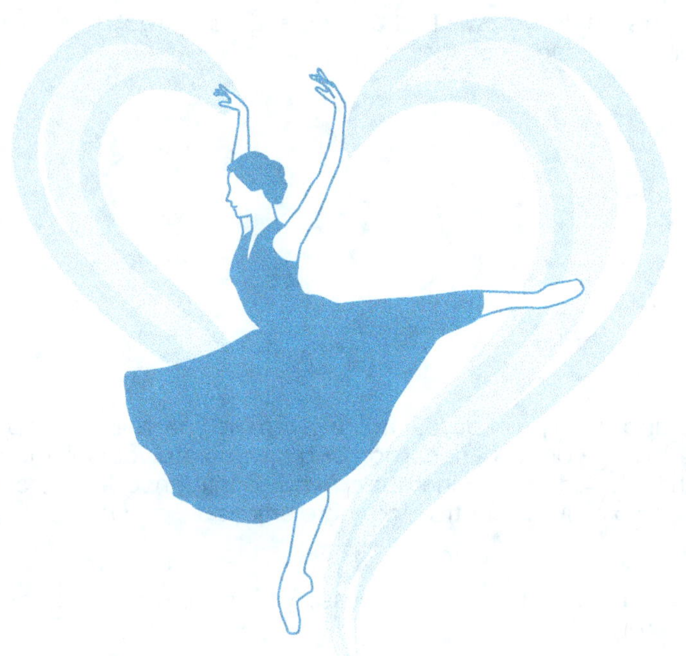

Avoiding Injuries

Stronger Bodies, Brighter and Long-Lasting Careers

As dancers, pain is a daily visitor and our bodies usually hurt. It's all part of just another day in class.

Dancers practice hard from early childhood and continue to work and rehearse for long hours until their career ends. We practice movements that require extreme strength, flexibility, and endurance, so how could we possibly avoid pain?

We've learned that we just have to keep going. So it is not at all strange that dancers usually don't give their body the attention it needs – even when it hurts.

Phrases like "if you can walk you can dance," "push through the pain," "dance till you drop," and "no pain no gain" are very common in the dance world. But these clichés are often misunderstood by both teachers and dancers alike. And taking them too far can put your dance dream in danger.

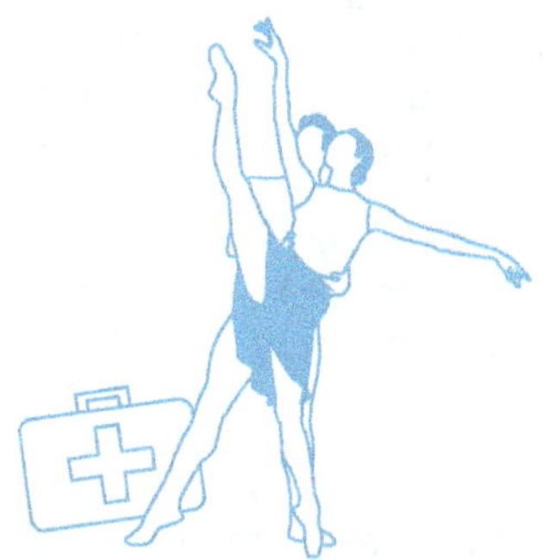

Consider these shocking facts:

Research has shown that 84% to 95% of dancers are affected by injury at some point in their career. Further, a year-long study of professional ballet dancers reported 355 injuries in 52 dancers; an average of nearly seven injuries per dancer in a single year.

Seven injuries per year! Injury is the biggest threat to dance dreams out there. Doing everything we can to avoid it is crucial.

Although injury challenges are faced by people in sports as well, dance has its own unique challenges that we need to be aware of.

Yes, dancers are unique, magical creatures! But you need to be aware of the specific challenges you face as a ballet dancer so you can protect your body and secure a long-term dance career.

Although pain is an indivisible part of a ballet dancer's life and no dancer can or should avoid it, a mindful approach is necessary in order to understand the difference between pain from hard work that will help you grow, and pain from obsessive mentalities that can lead to irreversible injuries in the long term.

A common misconception in ballet culture is the idea that without suffering you can't gain anything. Ballet dancers are often encouraged to keep pushing their limits, even when they are injured. Pushing through pain is considered a sign of hard work, determination and strength.

You've likely seen or maybe even experienced yourself, dancers feeling proud of pushing through despite advice from doctors or physiotherapists. Dancers often put their bodies in danger by pushing through their pain, fearing they may miss out on opportunities, or be stigmatized as "injured" by teachers, directors and choreographers.

Consequently, a dancer may keep their injury or pain a secret, and continue performing, potentially exacerbating their injuries. They may fall into a routine of taking painkillers, or dancing while being numbed with anesthetic or cortisone. But ultimately, ignoring pain is self-defeating, and can result in you spending more time away from dance and suffering greater setbacks in your career.

In the joy of this beautiful yet challenging art, we tend to forget that the body has its own limitations, and a serious injury can deprive you of achieving your dance dream and career.

So let's take a mindful approach that will guarantee our growth but also keep us safe from injuries.

Know Your Pain 

The reality is that you are going to experience some degree of pain in every class, rehearsal, and performance for the rest of your ballet life. And that is something you already know.

But you should never forget that dancing is a long-term game. If you want to have a long career as a dancer, you have to prioritize your health. There's nothing more important than your body. It is crucial for both your physical and mental health – and thus your career longevity – to understand and be mindful of the difference between exertion pain and injury pain.

While soreness after a workout is normal and can go away with a good rest, massage or physiotherapy session, persistent pain can lead to complications that are difficult to reverse. Let's look more closely at the two types of pain you must be able to distinguish between:

1. Muscle Soreness (Exertion Pain) 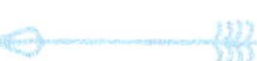

Exertion pain is defined as the pain experienced as a routine part of intense physical training. Basically, it is a physical discomfort caused by your efforts in dance training and performances. Exertion pain is a generalized ache characterized by muscle soreness, discomfort and fatigue.

Ballet is a demanding art that challenges your body by pushing its physical boundaries and creating muscle soreness. It is in this way that you enhance your strength and endurance.

You're going to experience this kind of pain after a demanding class, long rehearsal, or when you learn new choreography, because both repetition and new movements place your body under more stress than routine.

Exertion pain is usually dull and generalized. You are able to ease the discomfort simply by slowing down or stopping the exercise. In other words, you are in control of this type of pain at all times. Exertion pain can be a source of satisfaction, as it reminds us we are exerting effort and pushing our performance limits. This can increase our confidence and motivation, inciting positive emotions that can boost and improve our performance.

Exertion pain is considered "good" pain and the number one rule is that good pain usually goes away by itself after a few hours or days.

2. Injury Pain

As we know, ballet dancers have a high pain threshold and tolerance, and that often leads them to confuse exertion pain with injury pain. It's the reason many dancers end up ignoring injuries until it's too late.

A characteristic of this kind of pain is that it is not in a dancer's control to limit it. It is usually a sign of a more serious condition that could impair a dancer's health and threaten their ability to perform.

The following are a few characteristics that can help you identify injury pain. If you are experiencing any of the following symptoms, please visit your doctor and physiotherapist without delay:

- It is localized to a specific joint or muscle.

- It is sharp, excruciating and usually acute in nature.

- The intensity of this pain is usually very high.

- It wakes you up from your sleep.

- It lasts for longer than 48 hours.

- It's present before you start your practice.

- It increases with any exertion or activity.

- It makes it difficult to carry out other casual activities such as walking.

- It makes you shift your weight.

- You may take medications to lessen the intensity of the pain.

A skill that you should build is the ability to distinguish between exertion and injury pain. Note that this will feel totally different for each dancer, so you should focus on your own body – do not rely on the advice and influence of other dancers.

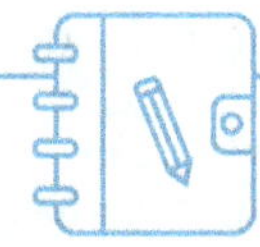

Good Pain/Bad Pain Exercise

Over the next week, evaluate how your body feels after each class, rehearsal or just before you go to sleep.

Try to categorize the type and intensity of your pain as good pain (due to muscle soreness) or bad pain (due to injury).

Close your eyes and do a full body scan, starting from your head and moving down to your toes. For each part of the body that you feel discomfort or pain, ask yourself the following questions:

- When did I start feeling this particular pain? Today? A few days ago?

- Do I have mild, moderate or severe discomfort?

- What type of pain am I experiencing?

- Is it muscular or is it located in a joint?

- On a scale of 0 to 10, what would I rate my pain?

- Is it different from the usual pain I experience after a demanding class?

- Does it go away after I get a good rest?

An honest evaluation will help you understand what your body really needs. It will assist you in identifying an injury in its early stages, thus protecting your dance dream.

Whenever you try to perform with an injury, you are putting your body at high risk of developing a second injury. So always think long term and be honest with yourself when it comes to evaluating your pain.

If you identify your pain as something more than exertion pain, get it treated without delay. The earlier you take care of it, the better your chances of making a quick recovery and returning to your passion.

Risk Factors for Injury 

While injuries are sometimes seen as an unavoidable part of dance, there are a number of risk factors you should be aware of:

Muscle Imbalance

Muscles work in "antagonistic" pairs. When one contracts, the other relaxes to allow the action to be performed. For example, in an attitude derrière, the agonists are the hamstring and gluteal muscles. They activate to move the leg to the back into hip extension. The antagonists are the hip flexors, or the muscles along the front of the hip, which stretch as the hamstrings and glutes contract. An imbalance between the length and strength relationship of these muscles can cause an injury.

Additionally, muscle imbalance occurs when there's a difference in size, strength, or tightness between corresponding muscles on opposite sides of your body. These imbalances can arise from faulty techniques or natural asymmetries.

In your ballet training, it is important to:

- Always be mindful and aware of your technique

- Stretch the muscles that you strengthen, and strengthen the muscles that you stretch

- Get frequent screenings in order to check any muscular imbalance to prevent serious problems from emerging.

Faulty Technique

As ballet dancers, we perform repetitive movements for several hours a day, almost every day!

So, the risk of an injury is very high if you are repeatedly engaged in the wrong technique. Remember also that an injury that occurs because of faulty technique is likely to occur again unless the fault is corrected.

It is important to remember the following:

- Always work correctly, with proper technique and alignment.

- Ensure you are being trained by knowledgeable, experienced and qualified teachers.

- Be patient with your progress. First ensure the quality of each technique and then push it to a higher level.

- Regardless of your level, it is often necessary and helpful to go back to the fundamentals of ballet technique.

Being aware of the quality of your technique will reduce your chances of getting injured and ensure your dancing longevity and success!

Become Injury Safe

In addition to knowing the risk factors, there are a number of other important elements that can help you prevent injury. Here are a few things to consider:

Positive Social Support ⟴————⟩⟩⟩

In ballet, as in any area of life, it is important to have positive social support around you. Ensure you have people in your life with whom you can share your challenges, fears and dreams. A 2004 Stanford University study found that negative stressors in ballet dancers' lives, such as worry and lack of confidence, led to an increased injury rate. However, they also found that this could be overcome by the presence of positive social support in the dancers' lives. Researchers also determined that ballet dancers who are taught general psychological coping skills experience fewer injuries.

It is also important to choose health professionals that have worked a lot with dancers and understand the unique aspects and demands of our art. Find a specialist that will not treat you like an athlete but like an athletic artist.

Unfortunately, most dancers do not enjoy access to specialized health care on a par with their counterparts in traditional sports. The response they receive from their health care provider is often unconstructive, or even discouraging. A 2012 study in Singapore found that 80% of university dancers surveyed felt their health care providers did not understand dancers. In addition, 43% indicated that their health care providers gave unhelpful advice.

A Good Warm-Up ⟴————⟩⟩⟩

Think for a moment about how your body feels when your muscles are not warm enough – or worse, when they are completely cold. There is a general discomfort, isn't there? Your body is stiff, your joints are tight, if there's pain it becomes more intense... The list goes on.

No doubt you already know that if your muscles are not warm enough before every dance activity there is a very high chance of getting injured. Warm-up prepares you physically and mentally for the transition from your outside life into the class or stage life. Always remember that a good warm-up is crucial for the protection of your body, and for the success of a workout.

Physical preparation

Living up to its name, a warm-up gradually raises your body temperature, priming your muscles and joints for the movements required in dance.

It progressively prepares you physically. Blood pumps faster, delivering more oxygen to your muscles. Your entire body warms up, and your energy systems become more efficient. This translates to a stronger heartbeat, deeper breathing, and the fuel you need to dance your best.

Mental preparation

It can be easy to forget that warming-up mentally is just as important as physical preparation. Dance requires high levels of concentration and mental readiness, and this can begin with the warm-up.

As you warm up, the focus naturally moves inwards. The worries and pressures of daily life melt away, replaced by a sense of mindful connection to your body.

You also become aware of any discomfort, tension or pain and are able to understand what your body really needs. This focus will carry over into your training to help you to improve every aspect of your technique and artistry.

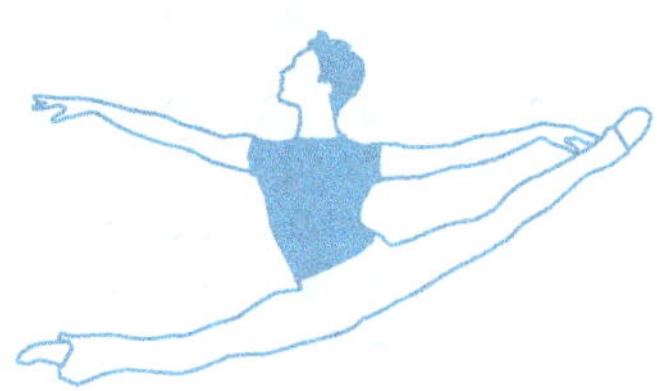

Stretch Carefully

Always remember that stretching is not a competition! So...

- Always keep your attention on your own capabilities and needs.

- Stretch your muscles to the point of mild discomfort.

- Remember that it's not about how hard you stretch but how often.

- Don't stretch too much when your body is cold. Stretching should only be carried out once the body's core and muscle temperature have been raised, as warm tissue is more pliable and elastic.

Vary Your Exercise Routine

Taking class every day without doing any other activity is not good for your body. It is important to engage in a wide variety of exercises in order to remain in peak physical condition.

- Ensure you are strengthening each group of muscles.

- Remember to work not only in a turned out position, but in parallel too. Repetition of the same movements creates muscular imbalances which can lead to injury.

- Level up your dance journey! Pilates, yoga, and cross-training are excellent ways to improve strength and endurance.

- Cardiovascular activities like swimming, cycling and other aerobic exercises are a great way to increase stamina, helping with the challenging schedule ballet dancing demands.

- Remember that aerobic activities can also decrease your psychological stress due to the higher amount of oxygen that is taken into the body.

Give Yourself Time to Rest

Most dancers know that getting enough rest after a demanding dance day, week or season is essential to high-level performance, but many feel guilty when they take even one day off. They believe their technique will fall behind and that another dancer will surpass them. This is the competitive nature of ballet. But your body needs to rest so it can serve you perfectly. It needs time to reset if it is to return stronger and healthier for you.

"When you work hard in class or rehearsal, micro-tears form in the fibers of your muscles. These tiny tears are what allow your muscles to grow – which makes you stronger. You have to give your muscles periodic time off so they can do this repairing and rebuilding."

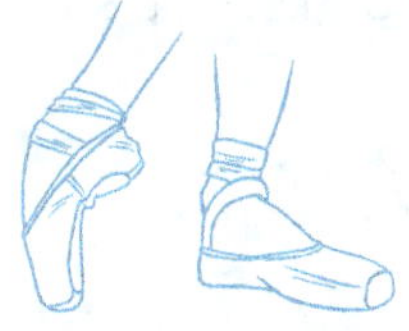

Michelle Rodriguez

NYC-based physical therapist who specializes in helping dancers.

Remember too, that mental rest is just as important. A ballet dancer needs a very sharp mind. You need to learn new steps, complex combinations and choreographies, and you need to do it fast. You constantly receive corrections that you have to apply immediately (and the list goes on). So give your mind a rest in order for it to be more efficient and effective.

Always listen to your body when it says: I've reached my limits! Allow it to rest properly! Always treat it with love and respect!

In the words of Natalia Makarova, "Because my profession is the body, it is a relaxation for me to get out of physicality and concentrate on more mental things."

Sleep, Eat and Hydrate well

As we've already discussed, sleeping and eating properly is crucial for your performance and overall health.

Sleep

Restful sleep allows your body to recover fully, repair and regenerate cells after training, reduces the risk of injury, and gives you mental clarity.

Nutrition

Eating properly can greatly increase your energy, focus and concentration. It will also help prevent injury and fatigue. Always try to work with a nutritional expert to keep both your body and mind healthy.

Hydration

As a dancer, you lose large amounts of fluid through sweat. So don't forget to hydrate properly.

The more energy you expend, the greater your fluid needs.

Replace Your Pointe Shoes Frequently

While a noticeable curve may sound lovely and desirable, a foot in an old pointe shoe is at great risk of getting injured.

Your feet need proper support in order to protect your muscles from injury, and dead shoes can't offer you that protection.

It's time to change your shoes when:

- The shank of the shoe becomes too bendy and cannot provide support to your ankles and arch anymore.

- You feel that you're "sinking" in your pointe shoes. This means that the toe box and wings (side of the box) have lost their support (i.e. the box is looking flat).

- You can feel the floor. This occurs when the platform has lost its integrity.

Push It, Don't Abuse It

Our body is our biggest gift. Push it, but do not abuse it. It is important that we treat our body with all the love, care and attention it needs. Learn to have more reverence and respect towards your body. Know your physical limitations and boundaries, and do not push it too fast too soon. Pay close attention to what your body is telling you, before, during and after exercise and do not ignore the red flags. Get those checked by a doctor before it's too late.

Try to open up and promote a culture of healthy habits in your peer group. Discuss the importance of paying attention to your pain, and create awareness amongst your fellow dancers about the stigma associated with an injured dancer in the ballet world. By doing so you will create a safe space for everyone to be more open about their struggles with injury and pain and take the necessary steps to deal with it in a better way.

Always remember, you can only live your ballet dream with a strong and healthy body!

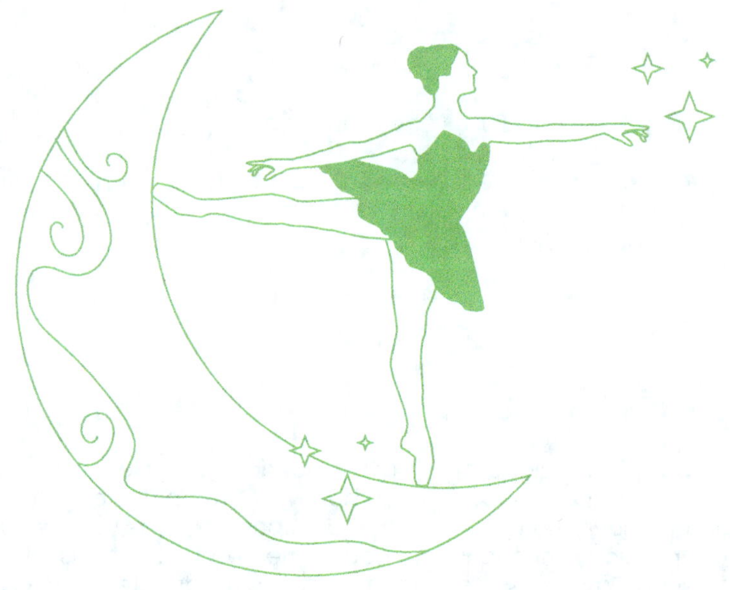

Dealing with Perfectionism

Brilliance Blooms Where Perfectionism Fades

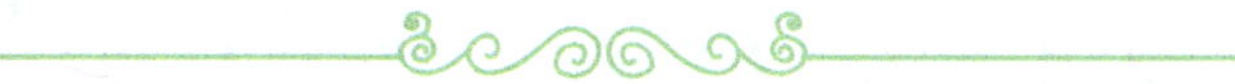

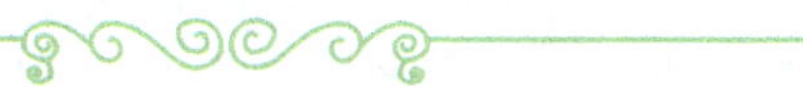

This is just one, simple example of the countless complexities dancers face.

That is the magic of ballet; It is an incredibly demanding dream that we love to give our heart and soul to.But we should also be aware that the uniqueness of this art is the most suitable environment for creating perfectionism.

Researchers have expressed their concern about the unique nature of dance, and have determined that perfectionism is very difficult to understand and treat among dancers.

And they are right! We are dancing in front of a mirror every day and constantly getting corrections from teachers, choreographers or directors. There's the struggle to get every single move perfect, the struggle for the perfect body and also the extreme competition that leaves no room for mistakes.

While dance is a domain where the achievement of exceptionally high standards is ideal, this struggle for perfection can have damaging effects on the quality of life for the most committed dancers.

Studies show that perfectionism is a predictor for depression, injury, and a host of other physiological and psychological disorders.

But what exactly is perfectionism and why do we need to be so aware of it as dancers?

One commonly used definition of perfectionism is that it comprises "the setting of excessively high standards of performance in conjunction with a tendency to make overly critical self-evaluations."

Researchers have determined that individuals with perfectionism often find themselves both plagued and paralyzed by their high standards and perceived discrepancies between their actual and ideal self. Their stringent self-criticism and attention to failure leads to all-or-nothing thinking, in which the only possible outcomes are total success or total failure.

When perfectionists fail to reach their goal, frustration and guilt causes them to dwell on their mistakes. As a result, they become overwhelmed by nonproductive, self-critical thoughts that can lead to a negative self-image. They see themselves as failures, and this loss of self-esteem can spark episodes of severe depression and anxiety.

Unfortunately, perfectionism takes away the basic purpose of ballet, which is to set your soul free by letting it dance and express itself.

Given the beautiful essence of this art, it's sad to see many dancers lose themselves in the trap of perfectionism. Striving for unrealistic goals of perfection instead of finding the inner satisfaction that comes through living one's passion, is leading to more stress than ever in dancers. This is not only ruining the essence of this beautiful art but also leaving little to no room for growth, creativity and inspiration.

It's important to zoom out for a minute and ask yourself these important questions:

What does it mean to be perfect?

Does perfection really even exist?

As **Mikhail Baryshnikov** said: ✩✩✩

"'My jump is not high enough, my turns aren't perfect, I can't get my leg behind my ear.' Please don't do that. Sometimes there's an obsession with technique that can kill your best impulses. But communicating with an art form means being vulnerable. Being imperfect. And most of the time this is much more interesting. Trust me."

Now we know the great cost that perfectionism can have on our dance life and how ballet can be a great environment for perfectionism to grow, it is time to see if there is a better way to reach our goals in this really demanding art.

There is Another Way

"Striving for excellence motivates you; striving for perfection is demoralizing."

Harriet Braiker

You may be thinking, "Yes, I understand that perfectionism is not good, but isn't this the nature of ballet; setting impossible goals and putting your heart and soul into it every day in order to achieve them?" And you are right. This is the part that confuses most dancers and makes them feel that there is no other way to success in ballet than perfectionism.

But there is another way:

We should strive for Excellence and not Perfection.

Although these two terms sound almost identical, they are completely different. To be more precise, they are the opposite to each other. We can even say that giving up on perfectionism is the way to achieve excellence. Excellence requires hard work, determination, effort and discipline, but in contrast to perfectionism, it tends to focus more on the process of achievement and not on the outcome.

Perfectionism is a belief system, not an action or behavior.

Consider the following scenario: Two dancers are both striving for the lead role in a production, but one is focusing on the excellence part by working hard, enjoying and appreciating the daily improvements in their dance. Meanwhile, the other is working hard to meet the high expectations that they themselves or other people have placed on them.

Same goal, same hard work, but different focus and belief.

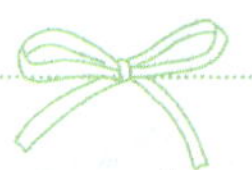

The dancer striving for excellence works hard every day, accepts the struggles they may be going through, and tries to do their best in this context. At the end of the day, they ask:

▷ Did I give my best self today? My best effort?

▷ How much did I grow today? What little wins did I achieve?

▷ Was my focus on the present moment as I was working on improving my technique, or was I drifting away into past thoughts and future scenarios?

The dancer striving for perfectionism works hard as well, but is fueled by the fear of failure as they try to serve the perfect image or outcome they have built in themselves. At the end of the day, they ask:

▷ Was I the best in class?

▷ Why didn't I receive a "bravo" today? Maybe I didn't try enough?

▷ If I continue like that, I will never get this role; I have to try even harder!

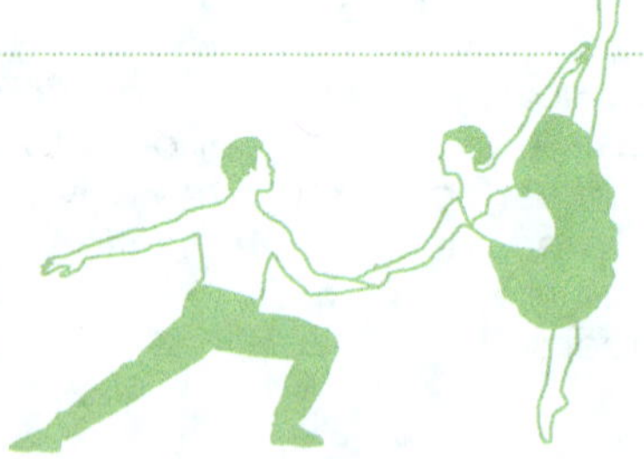

When dancers fall into the perfectionism trap they tend to treat themselves with less kindness and compassion. This keeps them in a constant loop of demanding more, asking for more and being more without ever feeling satisfied.

Remember, perfectionism is a black-or-white belief system; either I am perfect and get the approval or I am a failure. Even if you are a great dancer, you will never be satisfied by chasing perfection, as this idealistic expectation doesn't really exist. Being your best doesn't mean perfecting every turn or jump. It means always giving your best on any given day.

Perfectionism is always reaching for an impossible outcome in order to get fulfilled and accepted. Excellence, however, is broken down into little pieces that you can work and focus on with passion everyday while getting the pleasure and fulfillment of achieving them.

So it is really important to know when you are falling into the perfectionism trap, and to work on it before it becomes a problem.

Let's see how you can do that.

Are You Dealing with Perfectionism?

Dancers with perfectionism are usually dealing with one or more of the following feelings, concerns and thoughts:

- They are very concerned about what other people think about them; e.g. whether their teacher, fellow students or choreographer perceives them as inadequate or whether they like them or not.

- Their effort and intention are never enough. Results must always be productive and successful.

- They fear that they will be left behind if they are not perfect.

- They are scared to fail, and feel shame and guilt if they are not able to live up to their own expectations or those of others.

- They almost never appreciate what they have achieved and are always focused on achieving the next goal.

- They are very critical of their mistakes and have difficulty handling failures.

- They seek external validation and approval from others.

- They are motivated more by a fear of failure than a desire to succeed.

Tools to Overcome Perfectionism 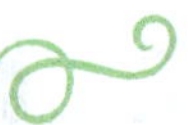

Dancers have plenty to gain from programs that enhance self-compassion and self-esteem. Such programs may reduce the damaging effects of internalized shame and perfectionism, be it self-oriented or socially prescribed.

By understanding the relationship between perfectionism, shame, and sense of self in ballet dancers, we can make changes that will enhance our own well-being and that of our fellow dancers.

1. Acknowledge the costs of perfectionism.

As you have already seen, perfectionism is not the key to success. In fact, research shows quite the opposite. It impairs your learning capacity and performance and gets in the way of your achievements. It is also correlated with depression, anxiety, eating disorders and addiction. The fear of failing, making mistakes, not meeting people's expectations and getting criticized keeps us from being happy, kind to ourselves and confident.

Perfectionism can lead to a dangerous and debilitating belief system. Due to continuous attempts to do things in a perfect way, one never feels satisfied. This gives rise to negative thoughts and emotions such as shame, blame and guilt because of the failure to live up to one's own expectations and those of others. Such thoughts can slowly begin to impair our performance and our ability to give our best. In an attempt to be perfect, we stop listening to what our body is telling us and what it needs.

Perfectionism usually leads to excessive training, which in turn leads to exhaustion, burn-out and injury. We also end up losing many valuable moments of celebration in which we should feel proud of ourselves, our efforts, progress, and achievements on our beautiful journey in ballet. This can result in lack of contentment and loss of connection with ourselves.

Perfectionism can also deter you from taking on new challenges that could help you grow as a dancer. For example, your perfectionism may not allow you to claim a place in your favorite dance company, a role, a promotion, or a spot in a dance competition as you may believe you are not yet good enough and that you need to work even more.

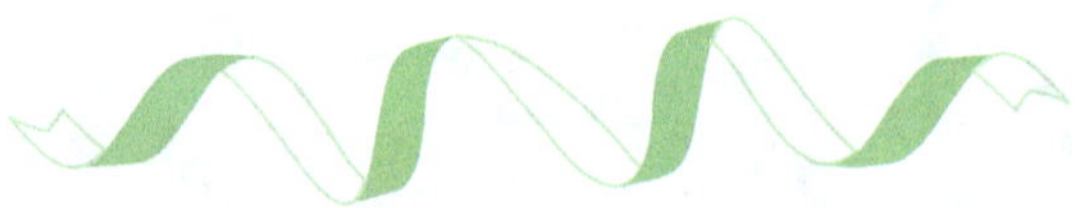

It also serves as a predisposing and perpetuating factor for a wide range of mental illnesses including eating disorders, anxiety, depression and insomnia.

Therefore, it's important to keep reflecting and keep our thoughts and beliefs regarding perfectionism in check in our ballet life, as the costs of perfectionism definitely outweigh the benefits.

> IMPORTANT: Continuously remind yourself that your goal in ballet is to strive for excellence and not perfection. Remember to give your best, but also to be kind to yourself and others!

This kindness and love will heal all the limiting and debilitating beliefs, and will set your imperfectly perfect self completely free. You will gradually begin to notice positive changes in the way you feel about this art and your performance.

2. Identify the beliefs that drive your perfectionism.

There are many thoughts we hold, consciously or subconsciously, that may be feeding into our perfectionist tendencies.

For example, many dancers hold the belief that they are "not good enough." This thought may lead to unrealistic standards and unhealthy ways of speaking to ourselves. Dancers who set these unreachable goals often end up anxious and exhausted, leading to reduced performance.

Constantly comparing ourselves to others is another example. If we regularly react to our own dancing with judgment and self-criticism, thinking about how others are better, then we are dancing to meet somebody else's standard of success, not our own.

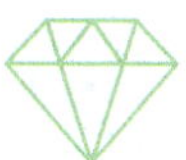

> Next time you are in class, pay close attention to how your mind creates a standard for your performance. Let your thoughts quiet down, and allow the body to express itself the way it wants to. When you notice a thought that feels unhealthy, let it pass without attaching to it. If it persists, ask yourself, "Why is this thought here? How can I allow my dance to come from my heart instead of my mind?"

3. Notice how feedback affects you.

Sometimes, a barrage of corrections can leave you feeling overwhelmed, causing you to lose sight of your passion for your art. Remember that negative feedback doesn't mean you aren't talented or not capable – even professionals must learn to cope with criticism. Handling negative feedback with maturity and positivity requires strength. It means loving yourself as you are and forgiving yourself when something doesn't go the way you hoped.

As dancers, we are always learning. Once you overcome one challenge, you'll encounter another. Learn from your mistakes, and be kind to yourself. Learn to handle criticism confidently. This will lead to a healthy growth mindset.

4. Engage in positive self-talk.

The importance of this tool cannot be overemphasized. So often, we speak to ourselves in ways we would never do with others. Be very conscious and mindful of the words you use when speaking to yourself. Instead of being overly critical, try to be forgiving, kind and encouraging towards yourself. It can greatly impact your overall well-being and your performance.

For example, if you keep falling out of your turns, don't let it define you or hinder the progress you've made so far. Your inner voice might tell you, "You'll never get it right." If this happens, immediately become aware of your thought and replace it with a positive one.

Go back to the Self-talk Tool and redo
the exercises if necessary.

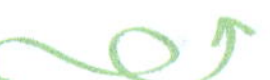

5. Don't compare yourself to others.

When we compare ourselves to others, we're only setting ourselves up for disappointment. We're each on our own path, with our different strengths and weaknesses, different bodies and abilities, and different ways of approaching this beautiful art. In reality, even those you believe are perfect will have their own concerns and issues. So, focus on you and what you have to give.

If necessary, go back and read the
Comparison Trap Tool again.

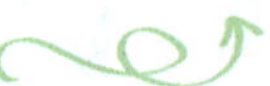

6. Practice self-compassion through mindfulness meditation.

Self-kindness eases the fear of failure and obliterates the need for flawless-ness. When you are kind to yourself, you have less fear of failure because you know that if you make a mistake, you are simply on the path of growth.

Try to cultivate self-compassion. Specifically, loving-kindness meditation can help you connect with yourself on a deeper level. Believe it or not, by improving your mental health and self-compassion, you are improving your ability to perform better.

As best you can, try to notice when you are being self-critical. If your mind is producing negative comments towards yourself, take a second to pause and breathe. Let go and start over.

By simply observing any perfectionistic thoughts, you can label what you notice. For example: "This is how perfectionism shows up in my mind. It feels like an unhealthy thought that doesn't serve me. I'm going to take a deep breath and let it go."

Mindfulness can be a life-changing skill and that is why you will find it as a separate tool later in this guide!

7. Reach out for support.

Silence and loneliness are the conditions in which perfection-ism thrives. Remember that you are not alone, and that you are surrounded by other dancers who are dealing with the same thoughts, the same struggles, and the same patterns. Don't be afraid to reach out!

When we're vulnerable enough to share what we're struggling with, we often find that others are dealing with the same thing. By creating a supportive relationship with even just one friend, you can stick it out together and cre-ate a mutual web of support.

If dancers started sharing their experiences with perfectionism more free-ly, we would all start to understand how exhausting and damaging this attitude is to our physical and mental health. Speak about your struggles openly – you never know how a conversation you have with other dancers might shift the culture in ballet.

8. Ask for professional help.

The above are some of the tools that can help us deal with perfectionism in our daily routine of ballet dancing. However, it's always a great idea to seek a therapist's help when you find it difficult to manage the stress caused by perfectionism.

A therapist can provide you with the support and guidance needed to assist you in dealing with and letting go of perfectionistic behavior. Mindfulness-Based Cognitive Therapy (MBCT) is also gaining popularity due to its ability to bring about improvement in perfectionist students. Go for the option that suits your needs and will help you feel your best about ballet dancing!

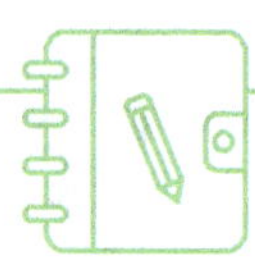

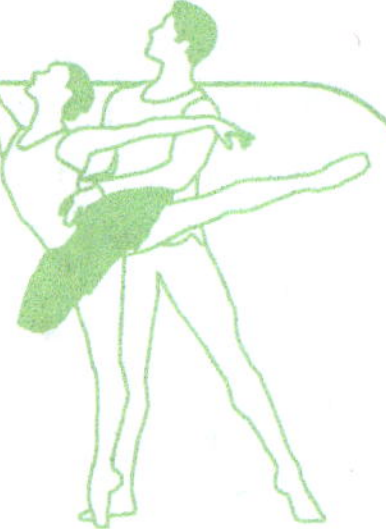

PERFECTIONISM MANAGEMENT EXERCISES

1. Affirmations

Write down, think or speak these affirmations out loud for the next two weeks:

- I accept myself the way I am.
- I am good enough.
- My failures cannot stop me from pursuing my goals.
- I use mistakes as an opportunity to learn and grow.
- I am proud and grateful for how far I have come.
- I love what I do.
- My passion for ballet dancing drives me to give my best.
- I do not aim for perfection but for progress and excellence.
- I don't have to be perfect to be powerful.
- Today I will focus on what is possible.
- I handle criticism with ease.
- I am thankful for all that I have.
- I love my body the way it is.

- I don't worry about things I can't control.
- I am going to do the right thing and give my best at it.
- I am unique in my own way.
- I feel the most confident when I do things out of love, not out of worry and competitiveness.

2. Evaluate Your Expectations

Write down the expectations you have of yourself. Evaluate them honestly and categorize those expectations as either high-standard yet achievable expectations or unrealistic expectations.

For example, it's not realistic to expect that you will never make mistakes or that you should succeed every time.

There is no way you can fulfill such expectations. Instead try to create more realistic expectations for yourself, as every time you achieve a milestone it will build your confidence and self-esteem, which will help you perform even better.

If this is difficult for you, ask a friend to help you with the evaluation of your expectations.

Expectations

.... Achievable | Unrealistic

.... Achievable | Unrealistic

.... Achievable | Unrealistic

.... Achievable | Unrealistic

.... Achievable | Unrealistic

.... Achievable | Unrealistic

3. Talk to Yourself Like a Sincere Friend

This is actually a very simple and lovely exercise – and you can practice it anywhere. For the next week, try to notice if any perfectionistic thoughts and actions arise, and write them down if they do. Write about how perfectionism makes you feel and what behaviors it triggers.

Example:

Thought: "I can't accept that I continuously fall out of my turns ."

Feelings: Anger, disappointment, inferiority, "I'm not enough..."

Behaviors and actions perfectionism triggers: "I should just skip the rest of class, there's no point in continuing."

Then write a note to yourself expressing understanding, kindness and concern in the same way you would talk to a friend experiencing the same situation.

Perfectionism Pattern

Thought:
....

....

Feelings:
....

....

Behaviors and actions that perfectionism triggers:
....

....

....

(As if you were talking to a dear friend)

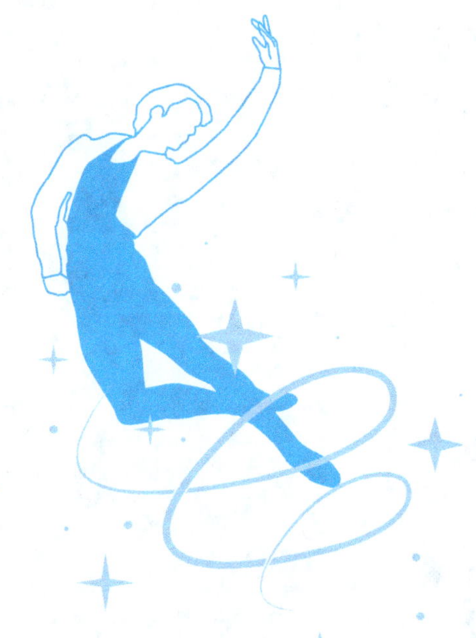

The Power of Visualization

See it, Believe it, Achieve it

Dance and Sport Psychologists use the phrase, "What happens out there is the result of what happens in here." In other words, your performance is often the result of what's happening inside your head.

> Visualization is a technique through which we can create mentally perfect images of what we want to achieve and feel, using one to all of our senses.

Ballet dancers cultivate a powerful mental image: their vision of the final product they strive for. This vision can encompass anything from a single, flawlessly executed step to a breathtaking sequence. It extends beyond just the physical movements, encompassing the desired quality, the emotions they want to convey, their ideal mental state, and even their interpretation of the role.

In other words, it creates vivid and realistic images in the mind, or "directs" a script in the dancer's imagination. The ultimate goal is for the dancer to enhance their technical, artistic and mental skills.

Visualization in the field of sports is widespread as its effectiveness is now scientifically substantiated. Champion athletes have spoken repeatedly about the benefits visualization has offered them on their difficult and demanding journey.

This technique is not as popular in ballet, but in recent years, more and more dancers have begun to use it.

There is plenty of research proving the link between mind and body. Everything you feel, think or imagine has a direct impact on your physical body. Just like everything you do with your body has an impact on your mind. Neuroscience explains that brain activity is the same whether you are visualizing an action or physically performing it. So as crazy as it sounds, the brain can't differentiate between imagination and reality.

Many studies discuss how the activation of neural pathways and movement patterns/sensations during visualization are so similar to those activated during physical performance that cognitive imagery is functionally equivalent to physical practice.

When you imagine yourself performing an exercise, for example, your muscles contract as if you were really doing it. The images that are produced in our brain carry stimuli to the muscles without us realizing it, since these impulses are very small.

According to the theory of symbolic learning, the pattern of movement is created in the central nervous system. The systematic mental repetition of a specific movement helps the pattern of correct execution of the movement be recorded in the central nervous system.

So if your goal is to perfect your turns, imagine yourself completing a flaw-less double or triple pirouette, always keeping the right technique in your head, from the preparation to the finishing position. Every time you create this picture in your head, the brain activates all the muscles that are re-sponsible for physically making your pirouette happen.

The benefits of visualization are not limited to physical fitness.

Mental imagery or visualization can also be used to strength-en psychological skills. It helps improve concentration, reduce stress and increase self-confidence. All these factors in turn help to maximize athletic performance.

Benefits of Visualization

Boosts Self-confidence

The dancer who envisions performing a movement or interpreting a role successfully ends up composing an image of themselves as a "winner." The dancer then feels satisfaction and other positive emotions that success creates. This boosts their self-confidence and motivates them to achieve even more challenging goals.

This is just one example of the extremely important relationship between mental training and athletic self-confidence.

Reduces Stress

Through mental imagery, the body becomes acquainted with those "difficult" emotions that accompany us in competitions, performances and auditions.

Visualization can help remove negative emotions like anxiety, stress and panic. Through this technique, a dancer can replace these feelings with pos-itive thoughts and emotions like calmness and serenity. Just imagine yourself performing calmly and confidently (or in any other desired mental state).

When the time comes to compete or perform for real, the brain will have already been "trained" to feel these positive emotions.

Improves Concentration

Our minds have a habit of wandering uncontrollably. During a visualization session, the dancer must create specific images which require complete control of mind and body. While using this technique, you must "see" yourself performing a movement or a set of movements thoroughly and with absolute clarity. This requires a great amount of concentration. So every time you practice this technique, your ability to focus and concentrate will grow.

TYPES OF VISUALIZATION

1. External Visualization

Here, you function as an external observer of yourself. You observe the whole execution of the movement and the general image as though you were a spectator. The sense of sight is mainly used here.

2. Internal Visualization

This type of visualization is kinesthetic in nature, as you imagine the way a movement would feel from inside your body. This makes it a more realistic form of mental imagery.

Research shows that internal visualization may have better results than external visualization, as stronger brain activation, greater somatic and sensorimotor activation and higher muscle excitation were observed in those who practiced it.

Try both ways to figure out which one suits you best. Then focus on whichever is most comfortable for you and practice it. Later, try the other one again and notice whether it offers you anything extra.

HOW TO PRACTICE VISUALIZATION

1. Be specific

Set specific goals regarding areas you want to work on in your imagery. For example, you may want to work on your turns, your petit allegro, your grand jeté or your confidence. Choose only one thing to focus on at the beginning. Once you're familiar with the technique, you can even work on an entire dance.

2. Ensure your technique is correct

If you want to improve a specific step, first go through its exact theory and technique in every detail. You have to be very specific and have the correct picture in your head. You can watch videos beforehand to help you build a clear mental picture of the movement.

3. Find a quiet and comfortable place

Ensure you will not be interrupted. Take a few deep breaths until you feel your body and mind become calmer. Close your eyes if you wish, or leave them open if you find it more comfortable.

4. Relax and start visualizing

Bring to mind the image of yourself and what you want to improve. Visualize the outcome you want.

This is not easy at first, so if your mental images are not clear or turn negative, stop immediately, take some deep breaths and restart. Then visualize again the outcome you want. Gradually, your body will learn to perform at your ideal standard. The key here is to pick specific things to work on in your mind and stick with it until those things become automatic.

5. Use all your senses

Visualize your dance performance in detail.

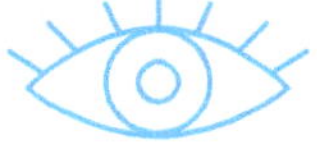

a. How do you feel?
Excited, happy, dignified, in absolute control of your body? Maybe you feel your body strong and ready to perform to the maximum, or relaxed and full of energy.

b. What do you see?
Are you in a studio or theater? Do you see the examiners looking at you and smiling? Do you see the choreographer enjoying your dance? Do you see yourself performing in front of a mirror?

c. What are you listening to?
The teacher praising you? The applause of the audience? The sound of pointe shoes on the floor?

d. What do you smell?
The familiar scent of rosin? The scent of your freshly laundered ballet clothes?

e. What do you taste?

The dryness of your mouth from concentration? The metallic tang of adrenaline before a performance?

The more detailed and specific you are with the images you create, the more effective this technique is. Make your image as vivid, bright and realistic as you can.

Make your senses the protagonists. Feel the excitement of successfully fulfilling your performance goal. The more specific and detailed you get, the more effective this will be.

When you are done, take some time to answer the following questions as they will help you understand where you need to focus more next time.

- Was the image realistic and vivid?
- Did I clearly see myself performing as I wanted?
- Did I see myself moving with confidence?
- Was I in a good mood?
- Was I able to imagine the whole environment around me?
- Did I use all my senses?

Visualization Tips

→ Start with just 5-10 minutes of visualization 3-4 times a week. Creating and controlling your images, especially when you first get started, can be tiring. Later, as you become more familiar with the technique, you can increase the duration. Do not overdo it though, because as with any type of training, it can lead you to become burned out.

→ Video yourself often when you are training or performing. This way you can have a clear picture of yourself and what you need to correct. When it comes to your visualization, you will be clearer and more specific. This will allow you to improve more easily.

→ Imagine a realistic performance. For example, if you're a young dancer, you shouldn't imagine yourself performing like a professional. This is a trap that can make you feel frustrated and want to give up. Imagine yourself performing the way you normally do, but incorporate positive changes that you are working on.

In the beginning, it is better to do your visualization in a quiet place before or after your rehearsal or class, or before going to bed at night. Later, you will be able to do it in noisier environments, such as a studio or theater. The more familiar you are with the technique, the easier it will be for you to concentrate, and you will be able to do your visualization anywhere.

Imagining yourself performing a step in slow motion is very effective. This way, you give yourself time to see the whole evolution of the movement clearly and in detail.

Gradually, you can increase the speed of your imagery until you can perform well in "real time." When you have gained more experience with visualization, you will be able to imagine in both real time and slow motion, depending on what you need most.

At times when you can't practice because of injury or illness, you can still keep up with your imagery sessions. An injury usually causes us anxiety about how we will overcome it and how long it will take us to rehabilitate. In such a situation, you need to approach both the injury and rehab with a positive attitude. Visualization can help with this.

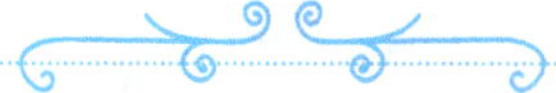

Imagine yourself perfectly healthy, able to move freely, without any restrictions.
Imagine the exuberant feeling of returning to dance.

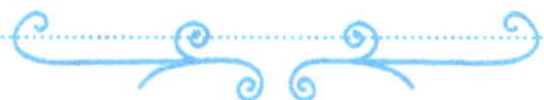

This will help you to maintain your skills during the recovery process, and assist you in overcoming your injuries.

Always remember: The only way to reap the benefits of visualization is to use it consistently in a structured way.

Repetition and commitment are the keys to success. Just like any other new skill, it takes time to understand it and see the results. Therefore, it can be helpful to set aside specific times and days in your week when you will do your practice.

IMPORTANT: This technique doesn't replace physical training!
Countless research has shown that the combination of both enhances performance.

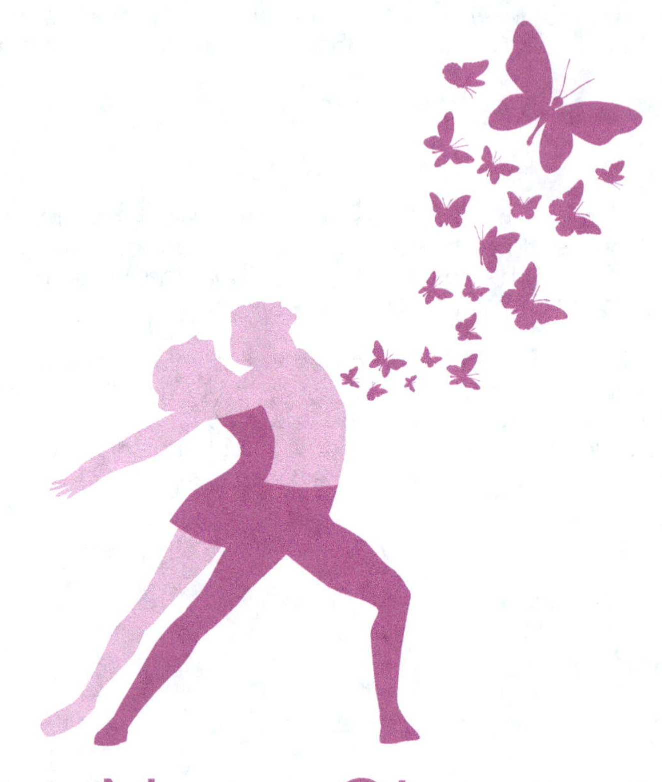

Non-Stop Motivation

Keeping the Flame Alive on Your Dance Path

Every dancer has days – or even weeks – where they feel unmotivated. And when we say every dancer, we literally mean all of them.

No matter how committed you are to dance, there will always be days when you'd prefer to just stay home, have a cup of tea on the couch, sleep a bit more, go for a walk, be with your friends – or do many other things".

The demands of a dancer's life are extraordinary. Many times, fatigue, pain or the constant repetition of the same routine can exhaust us both physically and mentally.

Also, our feelings can be influenced by so many other things: our daily lives, relationships, even the weather!

A dancer's life can get hard, making it very easy to lose our motivation, get distracted from our dance dream and start to doubt everything. This is the moment when frustration arises. The moment you may say, "I don't want to... I can't... I've reached my limits..."

These are the moments that test your true desire, strength and resilience.

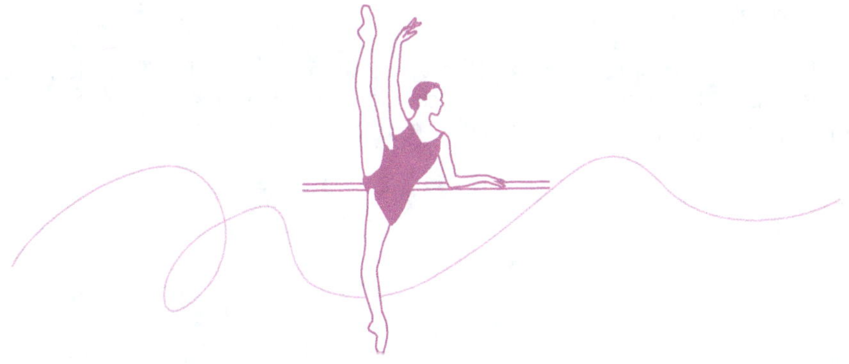

That's why motivation in ballet is so important! You must find the strength within you to work hard in the face of all the above.

Motivation will help you push through the toughest times during your training. It will also give you the courage to overcome any obstacles that might come your way. It will help you stick to your goals, no matter what.

Motivation is the drive within you which makes you put all your energy, effort and time into attaining a particular goal. However, it's also about satisfying something within you. That may be the sense of accomplishment, recognition, validation or fulfillment that comes from making your dreams a reality through hard work.

Through it all, motivation keeps you going when you're tired, bored, struggling or dancing poorly.

Motivation is your best friend when life gets hard, so learn how to increase it in your life in order to be able to achieve any goal set your mind to.

How to Boost Your Motivation

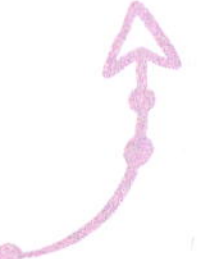

Visualize Your Success

In order to stay motivated towards your goal, it's important that you visualize it vividly. Daydream about it, and feel the emotions you would feel upon achieving that goal. Visualization is a great motivation tool.

On a tough day, reconnect with your goals. Close your eyes and clearly imagine the moment you achieve them. See the scene vividly in your mind, and feel the surge of emotions wash over you. Imagine the physical sensations of success - the lightness in your body, the exhilaration in your heart. This wellspring of positive emotions will fuel your determination and help you navigate any challenge.

Building a clear mental image of how you want your ballet life to look can help with boosting your energy, and can also be a strong reminder that every difficulty or misstep is just a small part of the process of living your dream!

Surround Yourself with Positivity

If you try to be positive but are surrounded by negative, grouchy or pessimistic peers or friends, it can be difficult not to be affected by them.

Similarly, your teachers should be encouraging, supportive, and non-threatening. A positive culture in class will help you accept feedback more easily, perform better, have an increased drive for training, and inspire you to give your best. Your teachers should be a source of inspiration and motivation for you.

Keep in mind that those with whom you spend the most time with have a huge influence on your moods. These people can affect the way you think, feel and act.

So, surround yourself with people:

- Who are happy and encouraging.
- Who value and support your dance dream.
- Who are proud about your successes.
- Who have their own dreams and goals.
- Who makes you laugh and soften your worries.

Maintain Your Health

Before you lose motivation and start judging yourself for not having the right amount of energy, courage or skills for reaching your goals, first kindly check with yourself to see if you are just really exhausted and drained physically or mentally.

Great motivation needs great health. You cannot be motivated and burned out at the same time.

Having a healthy body and mind is one of the keys to staying motivated, energized and focused on your goal. By not taking care of your sleep and dietary needs, your energy gets drained, making you feel stressed and unfocused on your goal.

Pamper yourself with a good amount of sleep, a self-care routine and a healthy diet every day and you will definitely feel more motivated.

Establish a Support System

Having a training partner is maybe the best motivation boost you can have. Training by ourselves makes it very difficult to keep our motivation high. A training partner who shares your challenges, goals and dreams can push you when your mood gets down, and you can do the same in return. Making a commitment to train with a partner is guaranteed to increase your motivation.

Be Your Own Biggest Motivation

Extrinsic motivation can be really helpful for reaching our goals.

Extrinsic motivation refers to a need you may have to impress your teachers, peers or followers, to win an award for gaining acceptance and fame, or maybe to please your parents. Extrinsic motivation comes in the form of rewards, which are generally provided by other people.

I guess all dancers like to get praised by their teachers, choreographers or directors, and maybe they would all like to be so good that they become known. Nonetheless, anything that comes from the need for external validation is always weaker than something that comes from a deep personal need.

If your desire is to improve yourself only to impress others, this can easily exhaust you and make you feel unmotivated. But if it is a personal choice to work hard and improve yourself because this gives you deep pleasure and satisfaction, it's far more difficult to lose your drive and inspiration.

If your love for this amazing art form is unlimited, if you can't imagine yourself doing anything else, if you need to dance because it makes you feel free, makes you happy, and brings out your most creative self, you will find a way to motivate yourself even in the most difficult and disappointing times.

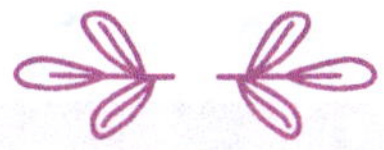

Dream of exploring dance and
unlocking your body's potential?

Yearn to express yourself and
become the best version of you?

Intrinsic motivation is the key – the most
powerful fuel for your journey.

To enjoy success and longevity in
dance, this is the type of motivation you
need to invest in.

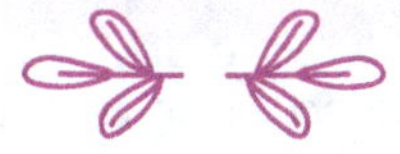

A great exercise is to create a list of both the extrinsic and the intrinsic reasons you dance and return to this list every time you need motivation. Sometimes an intrinsic reason will be enough. Other times, an extrinsic reason will give you the motivation boost you need on a particular day.

Extrinsic reasons may be:
- To make my parents proud
- To earn my teacher's approval
- To get a dance trophy.

Intrinsic reasons may be:
- My love for dance
- Enjoying the dance class
- To improve my technique and artistry

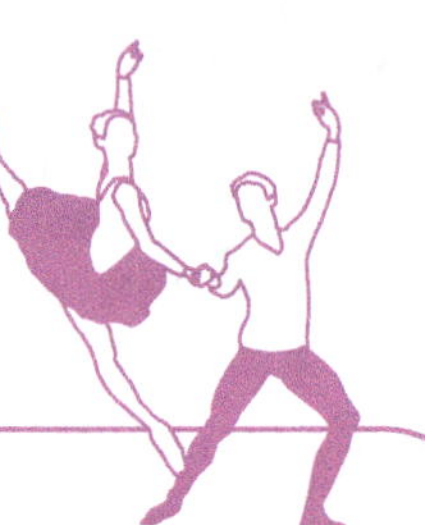

Extrinsic vs Intrinsic List

Write down your own reasons for choosing ballet as your dream goal in life.

Extrinsic	Intrinsic
....	....
....	....
....	....

Find Inspiration

Finding sources of inspiration is a great way to boost your motivation. Watch and analyze your favorite dancers. Read their interviews, learn about their lives and daily habits, the difficulties they faced, the secrets of their success.

You can also create in your mobile device or your room a small toolkit of motivation ready to be used when necessary that can include images of your favorite dancers, quotes, videos and photos of your own past successes.

You can combine all of the above in the following exercise.

The Motivation Vision Board: A fun and inspiring exercise that can help you stay focused on your ballet goals is to create a 'Motivation Vision Board'.

1. Gather Materials: You'll need a large piece of poster board or cardboard, scissors, glue, markers, and a variety of magazines or printed images. If you have any ballet magazines or programs from past performances, those could be perfect!

2. Your Goals: You have already written down your short-term and long-term dance goals. Go back to the goals tool and read them again, as they will guide the next step.

3. Find Images: Look through the magazines or online for images that represent your goals and inspire you. These could be pictures of dancers you admire, images of beautiful dance costumes or grand stages, or even words and quotes that motivate you.

4. Create Your Board: Start arranging your images on your board. You can create sections for different types of goals (e.g. training goals, lifestyle goals), or mix everything together in a way that's visually appealing to you.

5. Add Personal Touches: Use the markers to add any personal touches, like your own motivational quotes or specific dates for achieving your goals.

6. Display Your Board: Place your vision board somewhere you'll see it every day, like near your mirror or next to your bed.

7. Reflect Daily: Spend a few minutes each day looking at your vision board and visualizing yourself achieving the goals represented there.

This visual reminder of what you're working towards can be a powerful motivator on days when you're feeling low on energy or facing challenges in your dance practice.

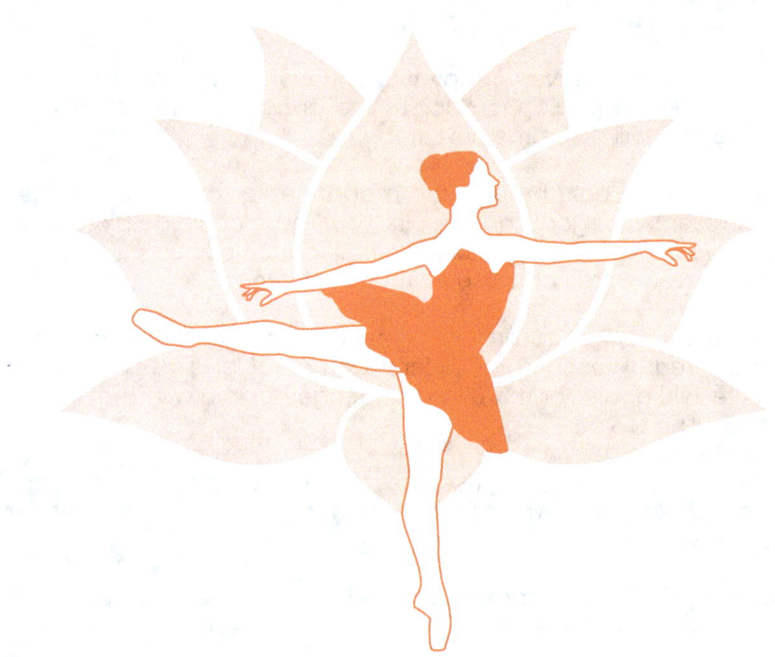

The Mindful Dancer

Be present, be powerful

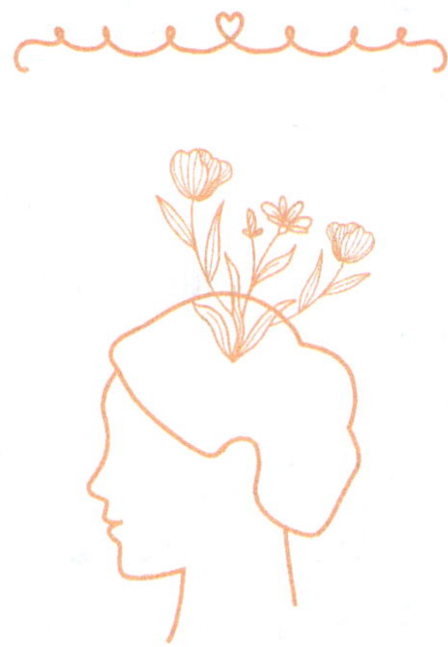

Naturally, we have many things to worry about. We dwell on the past: "Was that performance good enough? Why did I make the same mistake again?" And we continuously worry about the future: about auditions, being cast in the new production, getting a contract, and upcoming performances. Sometimes it feels like our brains are going a mile a minute with all these thoughts and worries – and not always in productive ways.

Also, dancers have so many distractions! These may include what others think about them (i.e. peers, teachers), technical anxieties, pain and discomfort during performance, stage noise and lighting, a drafty theater or uneven stage surface, costume malfunctions, things that are unrelated to dance (we are also human beings!) ... and so many others.

The physical and mental tiredness that dancers experience thanks to the constant demands of ballet, can lead to reduced concentration.

Therefore staying present is a dancer's greatest challenge. Losing focus, whether from internal thoughts or external distractions, can drastically impact performance. From classes and rehearsals to auditions and the big stage, mastering the ability to quiet the mind and channel all energy into the present moment is a key skill for any dancer.

Imagine: You're on stage, but your mind's stuck on a technical mess-up from earlier. Suddenly, the flow disrupts. Mistakes multiply, your expression falters, the character fades. Most importantly, the pure joy of dance vanishes entirely.

As dancers, we spend most of our time, attention, and resources on the physical aspect of our art. We train for hours, yet often overlook what's most relevant and can actually make us "better dancers" – our mind. This "muscle" – our mind – can make us stronger, better, and happier dancers, if we just train it properly.

In the same way you work on your body, you need to train yourself to be able to focus on demand. You must teach your mind to follow you in whatever you do, wherever you are, so you can always give your best performance.

Ballet thrives on present-moment awareness. Each movement and artistic expression requires a dancer to be completely in the now.

So how can we train our mind to contribute to our maximum performance and well-being?

Mindfulness is a type of meditation in which you focus on being intensely aware of what you're thinking, sensing and feeling in the moment, without interpretation or judgment.

Mindfulness is the basic human ability to be fully present, aware of where you are and what you're doing, and not overly reactive or overwhelmed by what happened in the past or what may happen in the future.

Mindfulness Benefits for Dancers 

Practicing mindfulness can help reduce stress, and increase focus, memory, and concentration; qualities that are so important for a dancer.

Mindfulness has been studied in a number of clinical trials. The evidence supports its effectiveness in many different circumstances.

According to Brent Anderson, PhD, a physical therapist who works with Miami City Ballet, mindfulness meditation can benefit dancers by calming down the limbic system of the brain. Also known as the sympathetic nervous system, or reptilian brain, slowing down this part of the brain can help relieve the stress of many hours of dance training, auditioning and performing.

Mindfulness is a superpower that you can build and always have access to in both good and difficult times. It will make you a better dancer, guaranteed.

Let's see the benefits that mindfulness practice can have for dancers.

→Increased Focus

If your attention and concentration are heightened, and you are focusing on the present moment, your perception will automatically spiral.

✓ You'll be able to learn new steps and choreographies faster.

✓ You'll improve your technique faster.

✓ You'll be able to calm pre-performance nervousness.

✓ You'll be able to get in the zone, the place where everything flows and happens more easily.

✓ Your confidence, positive feelings and pleasure will increase.

If you practice mindfulness, you'll notice that, in the beginning, your mind has trouble staying still. Your attention is drawn away, again and again, into thoughts, feelings, sounds, sights, smells – into anything except where we meant to put it.

By noticing and getting to know our most frequent thoughts, we untangle ourselves from the bind of automaticity. This process is usually a gradual one. We need constant practice to learn to bring our awareness back to the present moment.

Over time, as we train in noticing and coming back to experience, we can shift from a place of unconscious habit to a place of clearer seeing. This shift can be allowed to happen gently – one moment at a time.

The ability to focus and direct the mind is especially important when we feel stressed, distracted or overwhelmed.

→Acquire a Mental Balance in Your Dancing

Feeling overwhelmed by self-criticism? Loving-kindness meditation can help! It cultivates self-compassion, reminding you to treat yourself with respect and love. By letting go of perfectionism, you can finally appreciate your worth and efforts.

Want to improve focus and manage stress? Look no further than breath meditation. It helps you center yourself, increasing concentration and reducing tension.

Feeling disconnected from your body? Body scan meditation can help you reconnect. By tuning in to your physical sensations, you can gain a deeper understanding of yourself.

→ Boost Overall Well-being

The technique works by calming the brain's limbic system, explains physical therapist Brent Anderson, PhD. "The limbic system is where we get fight, flight, freeze," he says. Even brief meditation triggers the relaxation response, which boosts well-being, cognition, immunity and more.

→ Limit Injuries

A strong mind-body connection is a dancer's secret weapon. It allows you to become your own best critic, objectively assessing your performance and physical state. This self-awareness fuels a productive evaluation of your strengths and weaknesses, helping you improve without pushing yourself beyond safe limits. Through body scan meditations, you can cultivate a heightened sense of your body, noticing subtle details like tension, temperature changes, and even pain. This awareness empowers you to make informed decisions about your performance and well-being.

→ Feeling Fulfilled

True pleasure in dance comes from being present.

Being present means that your focus and concentration is set to 100%.
In that moment, there's no space for negative thoughts and feelings.
There's no space for perfectionism and criticism.
There's only you and your best effort!

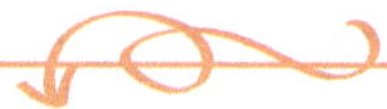

So, independent of the outcome, you will feel satisfaction, fulfillment and happiness because you have given your best self.

Mindfulness Is All About Practice

We can spend all day discussing ballet technique and the benefits of dancing, but if you don't go to class and practice, you will never reap those benefits.

Mindfulness is exactly the same. In order to reap the benefits, you need to sit and do your daily practice. Ten minutes per day is a great start. Consistency, not quantity, is the key to effective mindfulness. It is better to do 10 minutes per day than 40 minutes once per week.

Mindfulness Tips

a. Just Sit
Don't overthink it, just sit and do it. Guided meditations are a great way to start.

b. When
Choose a specific time in your day to practice. It can be first thing in the morning, at a break at midday, or before you sleep. Find what works best for you and add a reminder in your calendar or phone about it.

c. Where
Find a specific place where you can sit quietly without distractions. This may be a quiet room in your house, or somewhere in your class studio or dressing room where you can close the door and have some me-time without distractions.

d. Me-time
Don't let anyone or anything distract you from doing this every day. This is your time. You deserve it, so enjoy it.

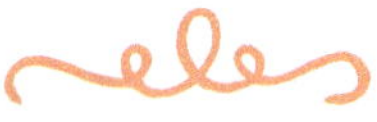

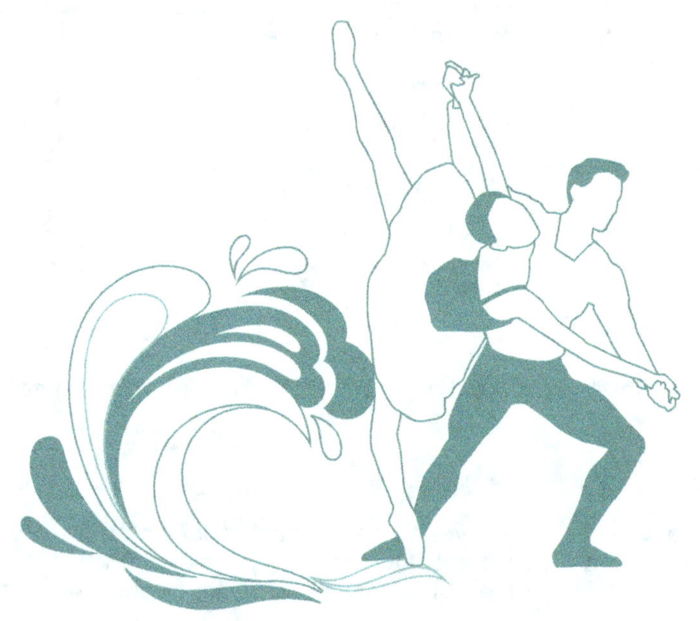

Dealing with Stress

Mastering Stress for Peak Performance

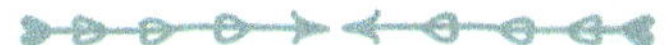

Stress is a natural part of a dancer's life. Long rehearsals, classes, competitions, exams – the list goes on. Balancing these demands with school, family, and friends becomes a daily hurdle. On top of that, the physical toll of dancing itself – the aches, fatigue, and lingering injuries – can push a dancer's stress levels even higher.

Remember, stress is personal for dancers. What stresses one person might not affect another. Don't get caught up in comparing your anxieties, focus on managing your own.

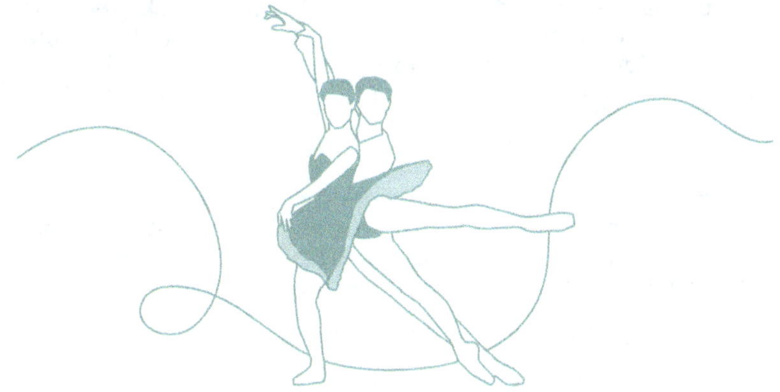

Stress is a natural thing in life and can be extremely useful when managed effectively. For instance, stress can give you the boost and motive to act on your goals. It helps you meet the physical challenges of dance by giving you the required energy and stamina. It also sharpens your thinking and focus, helping you respond to the intellectual demands of dancing.

But if stress becomes intense and persistent, you may develop burnout, as your mind and body crumple under the weight. Burnout is the result of a breakdown in your ability to cope with ongoing stress, demanding training loads without adequate rest, or the belief that you're incapable of managing the challenges you face. It can last anywhere from a few weeks to a few months or even years.

The Three Phases of Stress

Stress can be defined as a state of mental or emotional tension resulting from demanding circumstances. Hans Selye, the founder of the stress theory, categorized stress into three key stages:

1. Alarm stage

This is the first phase marked by an alarm reaction due to exposure to the stressor. During this reaction, the body's fight-or-flight response is activated. This triggers the release of hormones such as adrenaline and cortisol which help prepare the body for action.

2. Resistance

This is the second phase in which the body tries to get back to a state of constancy and balance after the alarm stage. Depending on the stressor, this stage can either last for a while or resolve very quickly without going into the third stage of stress. During this phase, we are likely to experience lack of energy, fatigue, burnout and poor concentration because of our body's attempt to adapt to the stressor.

3. Exhaustion

This is the last and most breaking point which occurs if the stress is persistent and becomes unbearable. In this stage, the body finds it hard to fight back the stress and can collapse as a result, becoming weak and tired. The stress can eventually impact our immune system as well.

Signs of Stress

The body's stress-response system usually resolves on its own. Once stress leaves our body, our hormone levels start to return to normal. But if stress is constant, we get overly exposed to cortisol and the other stress hormones disrupting the processes of the body. This can give rise to many different problems.

We are not equipped to handle intense, long-term and untreated stress, and it can have a number of damaging consequences. Therefore, it is important to know the signs of stress so you can pick it up at an early stage and manage it accordingly.

Some of the signs and symptoms you should be aware of
are mentioned below:

Physical Symptoms

- Muscle tension
- Decreased flexibility
- Frequent sickness
- Extreme fatigue
- Difficulty sleeping
- Appetite changes
- Headaches
- Digestive issues
- Teeth grinding
- Stomach pain, ulcer
- Profuse perspiration
- Rapid heartbeat even at rest

Psychological Symptoms

- Frustration
- Constant anxiety
- Feeling overwhelmed
- Poor concentration
- Social withdrawal
- Constant worrying
- Inability to rest
- Blanking out
- Lack of motivation
- Confusion
- Forgetfulness
- Mood swings
- Feeling unhappy with work
- Frequent boredom
- Addictions
- Overeating

Look at the list of symptoms above and answer the following questions
to assess your level of stress:

→ Which of the above-mentioned symptoms am I experiencing?

→ How frequently do I experience those symptoms?

→ Are there any specific triggers that cause them?

→ How long do these symptoms last?

→ Do they resolve on their own?

→ Do they impair my performance?

Stress and Ballet

Ballet dancers have their own unique challenges to face and these can cause high levels of stress. There will be plenty of situations in your dance career where you will have to deal with stress in one way or another.

The techniques and exercises below can be helpful to all dancers who want to manage stress more effectively. Stress is fierce, but if viewed from a broader perspective and addressed mindfully, it can motivate you to ex-cellence.

Types of Stressors in Ballet

1. Performance Stressors

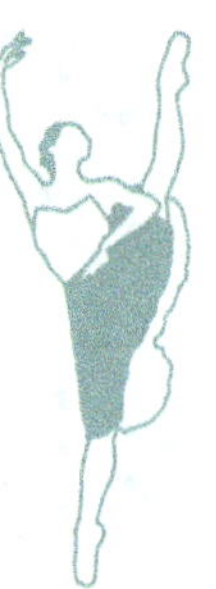

- Pressure to perform your best during an audition, class, rehearsal, performance or competition
- Technical and artistic insecurity
- Stage fright
- Long performance seasons

2. Personal Stressors

- Lifestyle issues or changes such as sleep disturbances, eating disorders etc.
- Financial issues such as low income or inability to meet your expenses
- Interpersonal difficulties with other dancers, teachers, choreographers or directors
- Inability to balance time between school, training and family
- Constant criticism about technical ability and physical appearance

3. Psychological Stressors

- Low self-esteem
- Fear of failure
- Poor organizational skills
- Excessively high standards
- Constant over-training
- Constant self-criticism
- Body image and physique concerns

4. Social Stressors

- Loneliness
- Unsupportive family
- Unfriendly peers
- Relationship issues

5. Other Stressors

- Career issues such as how many company positions will open up
- Position insecurity such as contract renewals
- Career progressions
- How the teacher or other dancers perceive them
- Getting injured
- Returning from injury

As we can see, there are numerous stressors for ballet dancers because ballet is a very demanding art.

It is very important to shed light on and recognize the sources of your stress. The more specific you are, the easier it will be to understand how your stress arises and how to manage it better. Try the following exercise to make it easier:

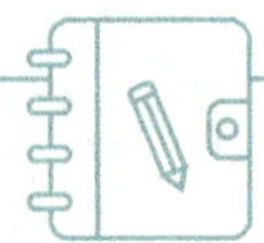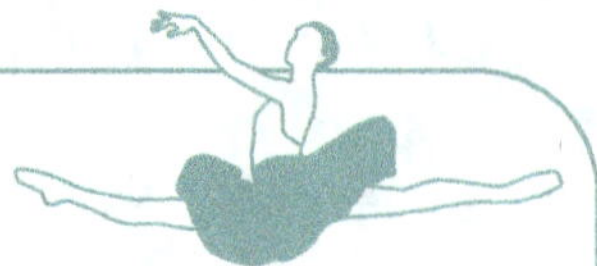

Dealing with Stress Effectively

For the next two weeks, observe which situations stress you the most, and how stress affects your body. Notice any symptoms that arise.

It is important to separate the trigger from the symptoms. Try to find the triggers that produce a stress response, and then be mindful of the symptoms you experience after the stress is triggered.

Example:

Triggers:

a. Over the last two weeks, I have been stressed out because the big competition is getting closer.

b. An old failure comes to mind again and again and I am afraid it will be repeated.

c. I was the only one in the class that received multiple corrections.

Symptoms:

a. I cannot sleep well and my appetite is reduced.

b. Headaches and constant anxiety.

c. This incident overwhelmed me, and I couldn't remember any combinations.

a. My Stress Triggers

1 ....

2 ....

3 ....

b. My Stress Symptoms

1 ....

2 ....

3 ....

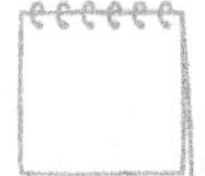

Dancers' Tips for Managing Stress

Dance is a demanding art, and stress can be a part of the journey. Learning to manage stress is a powerful tool for dancers. By developing practices to prevent, recognize, and control stress, you can protect your physical and mental well-being, ultimately leading to even stronger performances.

Some stress management practices are mentioned below:

Educate yourself about stress and its symptoms.

It's very important to be aware of the symptoms of stress. This will help you identify the symptoms and triggers at a very early stage and do the necessary work to overcome them. Also, just acknowledging the fact that stress can occur in your ballet or daily life makes it easier for you to accept and overcome it.

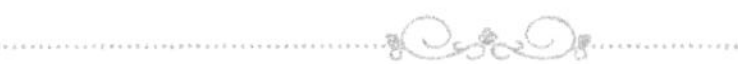

Do things that make you feel better.

Sometimes, a simple dose of happiness is all you need. A funny video, a stand-up comedy show, or time with your hilarious friend – laughter truly is the best medicine, offering instant stress relief.

Craving more? Explore activities outside of dance – painting, cycling, gardening, cooking – anything that sparks joy!

For a deeper recharge, consider incorporating weekly "me-time" activities. Think relaxing saunas, soothing massages, or calming aromatherapy. These regenerative practices will help you unwind and return to dance feeling refreshed and ready to conquer anything.

Remember, the key is finding what works for YOU! So experiment, explore, and discover your personal stress-fighting techniques.

Take care of your diet.

A healthy diet is essential to fight off stress as it helps keep our mood elevated and fresh, and strengthens our immune system. If you feel lazy, foggy-brained, disoriented or down most of the time, you may need to hydrate more, fix your meal plans, eat more healthily, or adopt an expert-approved diet plan.

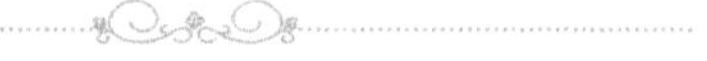

Take care of your sleep.

Sleep is the only cure-all medicine we have available – and it is free. Too little sleep is a main factor of increasing stress which can have a big impact on your intellectual functioning, reaction time, and motor control. It also increases appetite and makes you more vulnerable to over-training and burnout, which occur when there is an imbalance between vigorous exercise and recovery. In contrast, sufficient sleep helps you to bounce back from intense exercise or illness, fend off depression, and maintain a healthy body weight.

Meditate.

Meditation can be very therapeutic as it protects you from the effects of chronic stress and calms down your nervous system by decreasing the production of cortisol. This allows you to use oxygen more efficiently, normalizes the heart rate and slows down breathing. It also clears your mind and makes you more calm and creative.

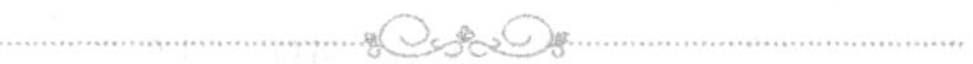

Create an anti-stress list.

Put together a list of things you know to help you manage stress. Whenever you find yourself becoming consumed by stressful situations, take a look at the list. By reminding yourself to do any one of these things, you will get better at coping with stress.

- I have a close network of relatives and friends I can count on and talk to.
- When I'm angry or anxious, I express my feelings.
- I do an activity that I find enjoyable at least once a week.
- I dedicate some time during the day to do breathing exercises and meditate.
- I ask for help when I realize I can't cope with the pressure.
- I recognize the symptoms of stress.
- I watch my diet and sleep.

Taking a regular look at this list will help you incorporate more of these into your routine. In turn, this will make it easier for you to manage stress on a daily basis throughout your dancing life.

Ask for help.

Feeling overwhelmed? You're not alone! Everyone needs a helping hand sometimes. Don't hesitate to reach out for support if things feel like they're getting too much.

Dealing with chronic stress? Taking a break and seeking professional help is a sign of strength, not weakness. It will equip you with tools to manage stress long-term, making you a happier and healthier dancer in the long run.

Cognitive-Behavioral Therapy is especially attractive for dancers, as well as athletes, given that thoughts and behavior have a profound effect on performance. Research shows that it helps combat a negative body image, reduce stage fright, and improve physical skills. In fact, it is one of the top choices for elite athletes who focus on mental skills training.

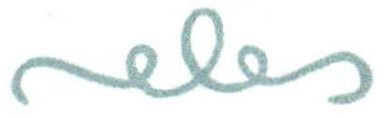

Your Personal Growth Toolkit

Ballet is a multi-dimensional art that needs a lot of training and dedication. In today's fast-paced world, life can become overwhelming, with information coming at us from all directions. This guide offers a variety of tools to enhance your ballet journey, but don't feel pressured to absorb everything at once.

Focus on What Resonates: Creating Your Personal Toolkit

After you've explored the different tools and completed the exercises, take some time to create your personal ballet toolkit. This curated collection is all about what works best for you. Having your own toolkit readily available allows you to easily integrate these practices into your routine, keeping you healthy, happy, and on track towards your dance goals. Think of it as your personalized dance compass, guiding you towards a fulfilling and successful ballet experience.

Focus on Quality Over Quantity: The 80/20 Rule in Action

Remember, the key is efficiency, not overload. It's better to implement one tool that provides significant benefits (think 80% of the results!) than to attempt ten tools at once and risk feeling overwhelmed and exhausted. This guide offers a variety of tools; pick the three that resonated most strongly with you. Perhaps "Setting Goals" will help you visualize your dance aspirations, while "Positive Self-Talk" empowers you to overcome challenges with a growth mindset. Maybe "Mindfulness for Dancers" offers a technique to stay focused and present during practice. The choice is yours!

Crafting Your Toolkit: Three Tools, Three Actions

Step 1: Identify Your Top Three Tools

Take a look at the list of tools below and circle the three that made the most significant impact on your journey.

→ Setting Goals

→ Positive Self-Talk

→ Fruitful Failure

→ The Comparison Trap

→ Building Confidence

→ Avoiding Injuries

→ Dealing with Perfectionism

→ Non-Stop Motivation

→ Visualization for Dancers

→ Mindfulness for Dancers

→ Make Stress your Best Friend

Step 2: Choose Your Action Exercises

Now, revisit each of your chosen tools and select one exercise or tip that you'll commit to incorporating into your routine. If needed, refer back to the tool descriptions to refresh your memory on the specific exercises offered. These chosen actions are the building blocks of your personalized toolkit. By creating your own personalized ballet toolkit, you'll have a set of powerful resources readily available to support your well-being and performance. Remember, the most impactful tools are the ones that resonate with you the most. So take some time, explore the options, and build a toolkit that empowers you to reach your full potential as a dancer!

Thank you 

We really want to thank you from the very bottom of our hearts, thank you for choosing to read this guide. We are deeply touched and thrilled that you're embarking on this journey to fulfill your dance aspirations.This journey isn't just about reaching goals; it's about embracing the process with joy and well-being.

You, the dancer, deserve to thrive on all levels. You are worthy of pursuing your aspirations with joy in your heart and a body that's strong enough to carry you through each step.

Remember, no goal, no matter how grand it seems, is worth sacrificing your happiness and well-being.

This guide, along with your dedicated ballet journal, is a powerful combination to fuel your dance journey. Remember: you have the potential to become an exceptional dancer. But more importantly, you have the power to cultivate a life filled with both passion and well-being. Now go forth, embrace the joy of dance, and chase your dreams with a healthy heart and a happy spirit!

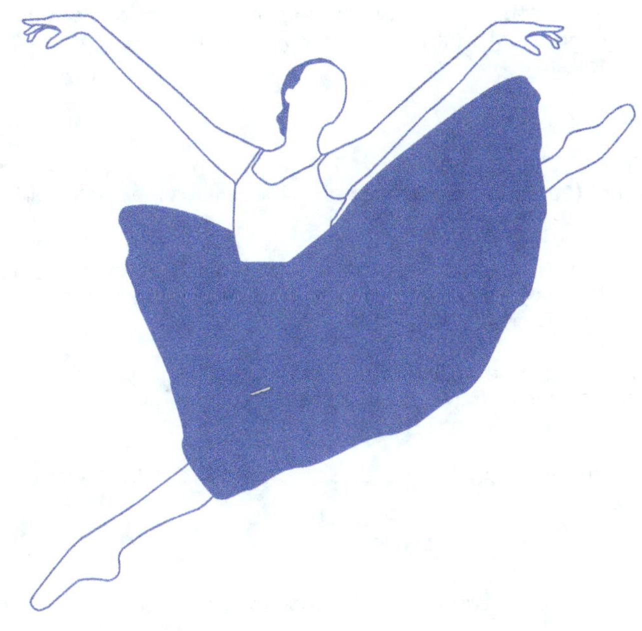

Live the Dream!

REFERENCES

Goal Setting

Locke, E. A., & Latham, G. P. (2006). New Directions in Goal-Setting Theory. Current Directions in Psychological Science, 15(5), 265–268. https://doi.org/10.1111/j.1467-8721.2006.00449.x

Taylor, J., Estanol, E. Dance Psychology for Artistic and Performance Excellence. Human Kinetics.

Taylor, J. (2017). Make Your Sport Goal Setting S.M.A.R.T.E.R. Psychology Today. https://www.psychologytoday.com/us/blog/the-power-prime/201710/make-your-sports-goal-setting-smarter

Self-Talk

Davenport K. (Ed) (2006). Dance Medicine. Physical Medicine & Rehabilitation Clinics of North America; 32-1

Hatzigeorgiadis, A. & Biddle, S.J.H. (2008) Negative self-talk during sport performance: Relationships with pre-competition anxiety and goal performance discrepancies. Journal of Sport Behavior, 31(3), 237–253.

Iwanga, M, Yokoyama, H, Seiwa, H. (2004) Coping availability and stress reduction for optimistic and pessimistic individuals. Personality and Individual Differences, 36(1), 11-12.

Newberg, A., Waldman, M.R. (2012) Words Can Change Your Brain, Avery.

Fruitful Failure

Dance Spirit. (2011) Fruitful Failure. https://dancespirit.com/Fruitful_Failure/

Sagar, S., Stoeber, J. (2009) Perfectionism, Fear of Failure, and Affective Responses to Success and Failure: The Central Role of Fear of Experiencing Shame and Embarrassment. Journal of Sport and Exercise Psychology. 31(5):602-27. DOI:10.1123/jsep.31.5.602

Taylor, J., Estanol, E. (2015) Dance Psychology for Artistic and Performance Excellence. Human Kinetics.

Building Confidence

Fogarty, G.J., Else, D. (2018). Performance calibration in sport: Implications for self-confidence and metacognitive biases. International Journal of Sport and Exercise Psychology. 3(1) DOI:10.1080/1612197X.2005.9671757

Taylor, J.; Estanol, E. (2015) Dance Psychology for Artistic and Performance Excellence. Human Kinetics.

Avoiding Injuries

Adam, M.U., Brassington, G.S., Matheson G.O. (2004) Psychological factors associated with performance-limiting injuries in professional ballet dancers." J Dance Med Sci. 2004;8(2)

Allen, N., Neville, A., Brooks, J., Koutedakis, Y., Wyon, M. (2012) Ballet injuries: injury incidence and severity over 1 year. J Orthop Sports Phys Ther; Sept 2012, DOI: 10.2519/jospt.2012.3893

Bishop, D. Warm up II: performance changes following active warm up and how to structure the warm up. Sports Medicine 2003; 33(7)

Clippinger, K. (2007) Dance Anatomy and Kinesiology; Principles and exercises for improving technique and avoiding common injuries. Human Kinetics.

Dalzel, J. (2014) Top 10 Injury Prevention Tips. Dance Spirit. https://dancespirit.com/top-10-injury-prevention-tips/

Deu, R; Greene, A; Lasner, A. (2021) Common Dance Injuries and Prevention Tips; Johns Hopkins Medicine. https://www.hopkinsmedicine.org/health/conditions-and-diseases/sports-injuries/common-dance-injuries-and-prevention-tips

Hamilton, L.H., (2015) The Dancer's Way St. Martin's Publishing Group.

Howse, J. and McCormack M. (2009) Anatomy, Dance Technique and Injury Prevention, 4th edn., A&C Black.

Hutt, K. (2014). Muscular Imbalance Explained. Dance UK. https://www.onedanceuk.org/wp-content/uploads/2017/11/DUK-Info-Sheet-13-Muscle-Imbalance-Explained.pdf

Quin E, Rafferty S, Tomlinson C. (2015) Safe Dance Practice; Human Kinetics

Russell JA, Wang TJ. (2012) Injury occurrence in university dancers and their access to healthcare. Proceedings of the International Association for Dance Medicine and Science Annual Meeting 2012; October 25–27; 2012; Singapore.

Russel, J.A. (2013) Preventing dance injuries: current perspectives. Open Access J Sports Med, vol 4, DOI: 10.2147/OAJSM.S36529

Russell JA, Wang TJ. (2012) Injury occurrence in university dancers and their access to healthcare. Proceedings of the International Association for Dance Medicine and Science Annual Meeting 2012; October 25–27; 2012; Singapore.

Russel, J.A. (2013) Preventing dance injuries: current perspectives. Open Access J Sports Med, vol 4, DOI: 10.2147/OAJSM.S36529

Simmel, L. (2009) Dance Medicine in Practice, Routledge NY.

Sturgenor, B., (nd) "No pain, no gain": The Psychological and Psycho-social Factors Effecting the Relationship between Dancers, Pain and Injury. Academia.edu. https://www.academia.edu/12914302/_No_pain_no_gain_The_Psychological_and_Psycho_social_Factors_Effecting_the_Relationship_between_Dancers_Pain_and_Injury

Tajet-Foxell, B., Rose, F.D., (1995) Pain and tolerance in professional ballet dancers. Br J Sports Med, March 1995, 29(1), DOI: 10.1136/bjsm.29.1.31

Taylor, J; Estanol, E (2015) Dance Psychology for Artistic and Performance Excellence; Human Kinetics, USA

Perfectionism

Burns, D.D., (1980) The perfectionist's script for self-defeat. Psychology Today, Nov 1980 34-52

Cumming, J., Duda, J.L. (2005) Demanding perfections vs striving for personal excellence, Dance UK News. 59. Winter 2005.

Frost R.O., Marten P., Lahart C., Rosenblate R. (1990) The dimensions of perfectionism. Cognitive Therapy Research. 14:449–468.

James, K., & Rimes, K. A. (2018). Mindfulness-Based Cognitive Therapy Versus Pure Cognitive Behavioural Self-Help for Perfectionism: a Pilot Randomised Study. Mindfulness, 9(3), 801–814. https://doi.org/10.1007/s12671-017-0817-8

Nordin-Bates, S. (2014) Perfectionism. IADMS. https://iadms.org/media/5910/iadms-resource-paper-perfectionism.pdf

Schmidt, R. E., Courvoisier, D. S., Cullati, S., Kraehenmann, R., & der Linden, M. V. (2018). Too Imperfect to Fall Asleep: Perfectionism, Pre-sleep Counterfactual Processing, and Insomnia. Frontiers in psychology, 9, 1288. https://doi.org/10.3389/fpsyg.2018.01288

Non-Stop Motivation

Taylor, J. (2009) Sports: What Motivates Athletes? Psychology Today. https://www.psychologytoday.com/us/blog/the-power-prime/200910/ sports-what-motivates-athletes

Taylor, J., Estanol, E. (2015) Dance Psychology for Artistic and Performance Excellence. Human Kinetics.

Visualization for Dancers

Abma, C.L., Fry, M., Li, Y., Relyea, G. (2010) Differences in Imagery Content and Imagery Ability Between High and Low Confident Track and Field Athletes. Journal of Applied Sport Psychology14(2):67-75. DOI:10.1080/10413200252907743

Holmes, S., Collins, D., (2007) The PETTLEP Approach to Motor Imagery: A Functional Equivalence Model for Sport Psychologists. Journal of Applied Sport Psychology 13(1). DOI:10.1080/10413200109339004

Porter, K., Foster, J. (1990) Visual Athletics: Visualization for Peak Sports. William C. Brown

Mindfulness for Dancers

Bauer, C., (2017) What Benefits Can Meditation Actually Offer Dancers? Dance Magazine. https://www.dancemagazine.com/meditation-benefits-for-dancers/

Blevins, P., Moyle, G., Erskine, S., Hopper, L. (2021) Mindfulness, recovery-stress balance, and well-being among university dance students. Research in Dance Education Volume 23, 2022. https://doi.org/10.1080/14647893.2021.1980528

Make Stress Your Best Friend

Hamilton Ph.D., Linda H. (2015) The Dancer's Way St. Martin's Publishing Group.

Kelman, B.B. (2000) Occupational Hazards in Female Ballet Dancers. AAOHN Journal 48(9) https://journals.sagepub.com/doi/pdf/10.1177/216507990004800904

Taylor, J., Estanol, E. (2015) Dance Psychology for Artistic and Performance Excellence. Human Kinetics.